Travels through
HISTORIC MEDICAL
EDUCATION SITES
of Europe

Travels through
HISTORIC MEDICAL
EDUCATION SITES
of Europe

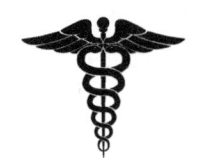

RICHARD HAYS

40

© 2020 Richard Hays

ISBN: 978-0-6488540-9-8

All rights reserved.
Without limiting the rights under copyright above, no part of this publication may be reproduced, stored in or introduced into a retrieval system, or transmitted in any form or by any means (electronic, mechanical, photocopying, recording or otherwise), without the prior written permission of the author.

Publisher: Forty South Publishing
www.fortysouth.com.au

Printer: IngramSpark

Cover, Design & Typeset: Imogen Brown

Cover photo credit: Rembrandt van Rijn,
The Anatomy Lesson of Dr. Nicolaes Tulp, 1632 / Alamy stock photo

TABLE OF CONTENTS

PREFACE 9
CHAPTER 1: A BRIEF HISTORICAL OVERVIEW 11
    References 19
CHAPTER 2: GREECE 21
    2.1. The Asklepion of Hippocrates, Kos 21
        Further reading 24
CHAPTER 3: TURKEY 26
    3.1. Bergama Asklepion 26
    3.2. Cerrahpasa Museum of the History of Medicine,
        University of Istanbul 27
        Further reading 29
    3.3. Topkapi Palace Museum, Istanbul 30
    3.4. Istanbul University Library 31
CHAPTER 4: ITALY 32
    4.1. National Historic Museum of Healthcare Art, Rome 32
    4.2. House of the Surgeon, Pompeii 34
    4.3. Virtual Museum of Salerno's Medical School 36
        References 38
    4.4. Anatomical Theatre, University of Padova 40
    4.5. Anatomical Theatre, University of Bologna 42
    4.6. Museum of Palazzo Poggi, Bologna University 44
    4.7. La Specola, National History Museum,
        University of Florence 45

CHAPTER 5: SPAIN 48
5.1. Old Quarter, Cordoba 50
References 51

CHAPTER 6: FRANCE 53
Further reading 54
6.1. Montpellier Medical School 55
6.2. Museum of the History of Medicine, Paris 57
6.3. Museum of Public Assistance –Paris Hospitals 59
6.4. Anatomy Theatre, Paris 61
6.5. Delmas-Orfila-Rouvière Anatomy Museum, Paris 62
6.6. Dupuytren Museum, Paris 63
6.7. Paris Medical School Library 64
6.8. Pasteur Museum, Paris 65
6.9. Library of the National Academy of Medicine, Paris 66

CHAPTER 7: ENGLAND 68
7.1. Wellcome Galleries, Science Museum, London 70
7.2. Oxford University 71
References 73
7.3. Cambridge University 74
References 75
7.4. St Bartholomew's Hospital Museum, London 76
7.5. The Old Operating Theatre and Herb Garret, Guy's Hospital, London 78
7.6. The Worshipful Society of Apothecaries, London 80
Further reading 82
7.7. Hunterian Museum, The Royal College of Surgeons of England, London 83
Further reading 85
7.8. Royal College of Physicians of England, London 86
Further reading 88
7.9. Florence Nightingale Museum, London 88

7.10. Great Ormond Street Hospital for Children, London 91
7.11. Anaesthesia Heritage Centre, London 92
    Further reading 93
7.12. London (Royal Free Hospital) School of Medicine
    for Women 94
    References 96
7.13. Alexander Fleming Laboratory, London 97
7.14. Bethlem Museum of the Mind, London 99
    Further reading 101
7.15. Freud Museum, London 101
7.16. Wellcome Trust, London. 103
7.17. Eyam, Derbyshire 105
    References 107

CHAPTER 8: SCOTLAND 108
8.1. University of St Andrews 108
8.2. Museum of Scotland, Edinburgh 110
8.3. Royal College of Surgeons of Edinburgh, Edinburgh 110
8.4. Anatomical Museum, University of Edinburgh 112

CHAPTER 9: CZECH REPUBLIC 114
9.1. First Faculty of Medicine, Charles University, Prague ... 115
9.2. National Museum, Prague 116

CHAPTER 10: AUSTRIA 118
10.1. Museum of Medical History, University of Vienna 119
10.2. Picture Archives, University of Vienna 121
10.3. Library and Manuscript Collection, University of Vienna 122
10.4. Sigmund Freud Museum, Vienna 123
10.5. Federal Pathological-Anatomical Museum, Vienna 124

CHAPTER 11: GERMANY 126
    References 128
11.1. University Museum, Heidelberg University 128
11.2. German Pharmacy Museum, Heidelberg Castle 131

11.3. Institute for Microbiology and Hygiene,
Humboldt University, Berlin..133
11.4. Berlin Museum of Medical History of the Charité..........135
11.5. Medical School Library, Berlin..137
11.6. Hospital Museum, Bremen...138
CHAPTER 12: HUNGARY 140
12.1 Semmelweis Museum, Budapest..141
Further reading..143
12.2 Golden Eagle Apothecary, Budapest.................................144
12.3 Burg Labyrinth, Budapest..145
CHAPTER 13: THE NETHERLANDS.....................................146
13.1 Museum Boerhaave, Leiden..147
CHAPTER 14: DENMARK 149
14.1 Medical Museum, Copenhagen..149
BIBLIOGRAPHY 152

PREFACE

This book provides an annotated traveller's guide to sites relevant to the development of medical practice and medical education in the modern western world. The focus is on Europe, because that is where modern western medicine developed and where there are so many accessible museums and collections. The perspective is that of a visitor from elsewhere, offering advice to others who enjoy travel and would like to explore some fascinating history along the way. The focus is on seeing and feeling, rather than just reading and imagining from afar.

I have included sites that I have visited, or at least tried to visit, that are relevant to the development of the profession and where there is something to see. I am an enthusiastic amateur historian who reads widely, enjoys art and seeks advice from other interested people. There is enormous variation in how some nations celebrate success in such a specialised topic, so while many sites are not really about medical education, I often found something of interest.

The book begins with the earliest significant site that I could visit, relating to the fourth century BCE, in Greece, and ends with developments in the mid-twentieth century in Europe, spanning almost 2,500 years. This takes readers from early Persian, Arabic, Jewish and Egyptian influences through to almost current times. The result is a rather eclectic series of commentaries based on the information I collected through reading, onsite observations and discussions with staff. There is a bias towards the English language, because I am largely monolingual, so I may have missed some sites because lack of knowledge or understanding. Almost any reasonable museum or art gallery in Europe is likely to contain something relevant to medicine. Sites are arranged in approximate date order, by nation and location, but can be visited in any order. Each site is interesting, and this book offers a sense of the relationship between different sites.

However, the book is not really about the history of medicine as that would require a focus on scientific discoveries. The book does not cover the developments outside Europe. This is quite an omission, as there are rich histories everywhere to understand. There is archaeological evidence of surgical practices from perhaps 12,000 years ago in Asia and South America. Finally, this is not even an authoritative account of medical education history – others have done that much better. References are provided for those who wish to explore the history in depth.

Because the book took several years to write during several work-related trips, maintaining information currency has been difficult. Details such as opening times and entrance fees change seasonally and some museums close for long periods for renovation. Access for those with disabilities varies and is often poor in older buildings. Website details were accurate at the time of publication, but readers are urged to check with each site before travel.

Despite these limitations, I trust that readers are inspired to visit the sites and learn more about the sometimes murky, but always fascinating, history of the development of an amazing profession.

Richard Hays

July 2020

CHAPTER 1:
A BRIEF HISTORICAL OVERVIEW

The history of medicine is, in fact, the history of humanity itself, with its ups and downs, its brave aspirations after truth and finality, its pathetic failures.

Fielding H Garrison, 1913

The origins of modern western medicine probably lie in the now long-lost cultures in the region bounded by the Mediterranean Sea, the mountains of Afghanistan, the Caspian Sea and the Sahara Desert. Archaeological evidence from the Mesopotamian Empire in 4000 to 3000 BCE indicates there was a strong culture of health and medical practice, including surgery.[1] The Egyptians left similar evidence.[2] However, this part of the world has been involved in so many conflicts that much of what was there has just crumbled through neglect, been destroyed or (more recently) removed to museums in the great European capitals, so there appears to be little left to see at their original locations.

We know some things from archaeological analysis about health and healthcare in the great Egyptian period as far back as about 3000 BCE.[2] Much of this is about the profile of diseases that were common at the time, although this mostly comes from the leading families, as their bodies were well preserved. Some show evidence of congenital abnormalities and others had endocrine diseases or spinal tuberculosis. Warfare and trauma probably drove the development of surgical techniques; there is evidence of splinting broken limbs, straightening fractured noses and amputations. Other significant developments were in eye surgery, circumcisions and trepanation.

The contribution to modern medicine by the Greeks is evident from the writings of Hippocrates (c460–c357 BCE)[3, 4] and Galen (129–199 CE).[5] Prior to Hippocrates Greek physicians were priests in a cult that honoured the god Asklepios. Known as Asklepiads, they worked in temples that were visited by ill patients. Illnesses were often seen as a form of divine punishment and the Asklepiads helped Asklepios "visit" the bodies of patients who were given sleep-inducing elixirs in the temples. If Asklepios willed it, patients awoke free of their illnesses. The assistants to the Asklepiads gradually developed their own more scientific-rational approach to diagnosing illness by bedside observation. They recognised that the brain was an important organ and are credited with the development of what might be the first medical school in about 700 BCE. The location was the port of Knidos, on the south-east Mediterranean coast of what is now Turkey.

Hippocrates lived at a time of great Greek philosophers and developed a different philosophical approach to understanding health. He travelled extensively, pondering the meaning of health, and further separated religion from medicine. He appears to have blended concepts from Arab and Jewish medical practices into his own learning. Illness was seen as an imbalance in the four humours (yellow bile, blood, phlegm and black bile), and that these were influenced by the four qualities (hot, dry, cold and wet), the four ages of man, the four temperaments (choleric, sanguine, phlegmatic and melancholic) and the four elements (earth, water, air and fire). Balance, and therefore health, could be restored through altering these individual contributors.

Hippocratic medicine was based on observation of patients and reasoning with those observations. His greatest contribution was probably his detailed – and in many cases still accurate – description of presentations of illnesses and diseases, a textbook of surgery and his long list of medical aphorisms to guide practice. An example of his aphorisms is "food when taken in greater quantities than nature requires, causes disease".[4] Many still make sense today as a set of "rules" that help make diagnoses and guide healthier lives. These are listed in treatises that were written over several decades, although Hippocrates was almost certainly not the sole author. The island of Kos, Hippocrates' birthplace and home, had one of the larger and more prestigious Asklepions that became famous for its medical school. Here physicians were trained in the Hippocratic tradition by what we now recognise as an apprenticeship model.

What Hippocrates is remembered most for, however, is his approach to medical practice that saw high value given to honesty and dignity of the physician. Some of his statements on medical ethics remain in use today. The Hippocratic Oath honours this particular man, but it probably reflects the views and contributions of several people over a few centuries. Variations of this oath are recited by medical graduates in many parts of the world.

The next great development in medical education took place in Alexandria at the mouth of the Nile River, where a medical school developed around 332 BCE.[6] Alexandria was a major site of Arab scholarship, particularly in pre-Islamic times, and was the site of perhaps the largest library in the world at the time, containing a vast collection of scrolls. Initially two medical schools were established, probably because of the library and its attraction to scholars, and

CHAPTER 1

their founding fathers were Kos-educated physicians – Herophilos and Erasistratos, who made advances in understanding neuroanatomy. The Alexandria schools played a dominant role in medical education for about 300 years, although they lasted in some form until about the seventh century CE. The focus of development gradually moved to Rome as the Egyptian and Greek Empires faded. The Roman Empire gained the ascendancy and absorbed the expertise and exotic influences of those conquered civilisations. Alexandria has been destroyed many times since its prominence, and nothing remains of the original library and associated places of scholarship, although a memorial to the library has recently been constructed near the port.

This is where Galen enters the picture.[5,6] He was by no means the first Greek physician to move to Rome, but he was the most influential. Born into a wealthy Greek family near Pergamon, now the Turkish city of Bergama (not far from Knidos and Kos), he developed an early interest in medicine and healing, initially heavily influenced by the large Asklepiad traditions promulgated in the nearby famous Asklepion of Pergamon. He was trained in a Hippocratic school and travelled widely before settling in Rome, working as personal physician to the Emperor Marcus Aurelius for most of his life. Greek philosophy and medicine were highly regarded in Rome, where the educated could speak and write Greek as well as Latin.

Galen's greatest contributions were made during his Roman period.[7] He developed the humoural theory of medicine further and added a new dimension, improving the understanding of anatomy and physiology through dissection of animals. Human dissection was banned in Rome, although dissection of war casualties was tolerated on the Roman front in Germany, so Galen used pigs, dogs and primates. Despite some inaccuracies that probably resulted from his primarily nonhuman dissection, his definitive textbook on anatomy was the standard resource for over a thousand years, until human dissection became established in the fifteenth century. He also made contributions to understanding of hygiene, exercise, illness prevention and plant therapeutics, and wrote a textbook on pathology. His thinking had a profound influence on medical practice and education for several centuries.

In most respects Roman medicine was Greek medicine, with a blend of other influences. This was a logical direction as Italy was great trading nation, with regular maritime contact with the Greek, Arab and Jewish communities. What we now call the Latin tradition of medicine emerged from a combination of those influences, some local innovation and the wealth to support development. The two most significant Roman contributions to health both related more to Roman engineering and organisational skills than individual brilliance. The first was the construction of public infrastructure to provide clean water for drinking and bathing, and for sewage disposal. The second was the development of military treatment posts, which in turn became hospitals.[8]

Medical practice appears to have developed more slowly over the next few centuries, in parallel with the decline of the Roman Empire and the instability associated with the prolonged feudal warring across most of Europe. There were several different philosophical approaches, and tensions existed between their practitioners. Some used numerology as an aid to diagnosis and treatment. Astrology was popular, as it had a kind of rationale that was appealing to theorists, particularly the early Arabic and Aristotelian physicians. Complex geometric measurements were used to diagnose ("celestial anatomy") and to predict the outcome of treatment. Popular belief held that right and left sides of the body held meaning, particularly for gender-related health issues.

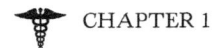 CHAPTER 1

Uroscopy was also commonly used to diagnose – some were brave enough to examine urine without taking a history or laying eyes on the patient – and most disorders were treated by bleeding.

Religious ideology underpinned medical thinking. The form of religion varied depending on location, and the development of medicine followed the development and spread of Judaism, Christianity and Islam, and the battles between them. Diseases were often viewed as retribution from God for some sin, so successful medical treatment was a gift from God; doctors were born, rather than made. Most of the leading physicians are remembered as much for their broader writings on philosophy and religion as for their contributions to medicine.

The next major development was the arrival of Islamic medicine, which developed primarily from earlier Arab and Jewish traditions. The Islamic Empire became vast, stretching from Persia in the east to Spain in the west. Two main cultural and educational centres developed as the "capitals" of the eastern and western caliphates, the first in Baghdad (east), the other in Cordoba in southern Spain (west).[9] Both centres are reputed to have had large libraries, schools and mosques; both centres produced outstanding scholars, philosophers and physicians.

One outstanding Islamic philosopher and physician was al-Zuwhahiri, also known in the Islamic world as Ibn Sina, and to others as Avicenna (980–1037). He was born in Persia and lived most of his life in the western caliphate, where he led the blending of Aristotelian philosophy into Arab medicine. He was a great thinker and philosopher in most aspects of religion and life. Because the healing arts were seen as an approach to life that included living well and piously, his writings include aspects of medicine. At times he was a medical practitioner, personally caring for the sick.

One of his more noted works is a cardiac pharmacopoeia.[9] This has recently been translated into English and makes interesting reading. He was heavily influenced by the "four humours" theory and classified herbs, minerals and other natural products by their capacity to influence the humours. This particular tract includes descriptions of both the raw ingredients (such as coral, amber, coriander and mint) and recipes for combinations of these to form oral or topical drugs to strengthen the heart. The list of maladies makes little sense in the light of modern cardiology, but there may have been a pharmacological effect. However, it is for his contributions to medical education that he is most remembered. He brought to Arab medicine the Greek medical traditions, including the work of Galen and Hippocrates and their great textbooks. He taught at a medical school or Madrassa in Isfahan and wrote his famous *Canon of Medicine*.

Later the strength of Islamic medical development moved to the western caliphate in southern Spain, this time with a series of famed Islamic scholars (Averroes was the most prominent, and perhaps as famous as Avicenna) and, perhaps oddly amidst wars between religions, the renowned Jewish scholar Maimonides.[10, 11, 12] Here were also translations of original Greek manuscripts by Hippocrates and Galen. It is a fact deserving of wider recognition that Islamic medicine kept many of these great manuscripts safe at a time that the Roman Empire was disintegrating, and many cultural treasures were lost. Many of the later Latin copies of these books were re-translated from Arabic versions.

The next phase of the development of western medical education coincides with the emergence of Christianity as the dominant religion in southern Europe and the re-conceptualisation of education that formed the basis of the modern university. These centres of education were closely linked to (and usually run by) the Catholic Church for the education of small numbers of clerics, some of whom became physicians. The curriculum was mostly Christian philosophy; the clerics wrote by hand and collected books to create reference libraries. Gradually the concept of the educated, rational doctor emerged, and the path of physician education developed. Medical thinking was dominated by belief in astrology, imbalance of the humours, prayer and herbs. However, early writings refer often to something like what we now call the placebo effect, whereby treatments were instituted with great confidence but little expectation of success, perhaps to make the doctor appear to be bold, brave and clever.

Around this time a revolutionary development in medical education occurred – the introduction of human dissection as a means of understanding and teaching about human health. Human dissection was not permitted under either Christianity or Islam, and so the spread of human dissection in medical schools almost parallels the spread of secularism, or at least liberalism within the Christian church, in European universities. Although not the originators of human dissection, the Italian medical schools institutionalised the teaching of anatomy through either dissection or the manufacture of remarkably lifelike wax models – perhaps the original simulation in medical education.

Medical education slowly spread from Italy along the Mediterranean coast of what is now France, to Montpellier and Toulouse, and then up through France to Paris and beyond. Paris enjoyed a period of cultural dominance and Parisian disciples then spread modern medical education to Britain, German-speaking Europe, the low countries and Scandinavia. These few centres remained the major producers of medical graduates until the next major expansion in the eighteenth and nineteenth centuries, when medical education expanded as doctors offered their services to a larger proportion of the population, rather than just to wealthy patrons. Amidst a period of European colonisation of the "new world", European-style medical schools were established in the Americas and Australasia. This phase of expansion also saw the growth in specialisation of the profession, as knowledge expanded beyond the scope of individual practitioners. Some of these specialties emerged from within the existing medical profession, while others came from outside that field, amidst amazing political struggles. This book is mostly about these more recent, fascinating developments, partly because of the availability of documents and accessibility of sites to visit.

References

1. Haeger, K. *An Illustrated History of Surgery.* Harold Stark Medical, London, 1989.

2. Filer, J. *Egyptian Bookshelf: Disease.* British Museum Press, London, 1995.

3. Chadwick, J. and Mann, W.N. *The Medical Works of Hippocrates.* Blackwell Scientific Publications, Oxford, 1950.

4. Coar, Thomas, translator. *The Aphorisms of Hippocrates.* 1822. Reprint Classics of Medicine Library, Gryphon Editions, Birmingham, Alabama, 1995.

5. Sarton, George. *Galen of Pergamon.* University of Kansas Press, Lawrence, Kansas, 1954.

6. Puschmann, T. and Hare, E.H. *A History of Medical Education.* [Translated and edited by E.H. Hare] Facsimile of 1891 ed. Hafner, New York, 1966.

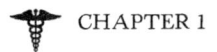 CHAPTER 1

7. Guthrie, D. *A History of Medicine.* Thomas Nelson and Sons, London, 1945. Reprinted 1960.

8. Singer, C. and Underwood, E.A. *A Short History of Medicine.* 2nd ed., Oxford University Press, London, 1962.

9. Hameed, H.A. and Avicenna. *Avicenna's Tract on Cardiac Drugs and Essays on Arab Cardiotherapy.* Hamdard Foundation Press, Karachi, 1983.

10. Ead, Hamed A. *Averroes as a Physician.* www.levity.com/alchemy/islam21.html

11. Shapiro, John. *The Jewish 100. A Ranking of the Most Influential Jews of All Time.* Citadel Press, New York, 1994.

12. *Encyclopaedia Judaica.* Encyclopaedia Judaica; Macmillan Jerusalem, 1971.

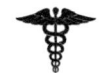

CHAPTER 2:
GREECE

Greece is the site of what most people in the western world think of as the beginning of modern medicine. That is of course a difficult judgement to make, but it was certainly the country that produced some of the greatest early medical philosophers and practitioners, some of whom carefully recorded their ideas. At the time Greece was much larger than it is now, occupying much of western Turkey, and reaching into what is now called the Middle East. Much of what we call Greek medicine in fact had earlier origins, with strong influences from Arab and Jewish medicine, which in themselves were developments of earlier ideas and practices. Perhaps one of the more remarkable features of the early Greek physicians was that they were better at marketing their ideas, because Greek medicine was the major early influence on Roman and Islamic medicine. For the purposes of this book, Greece is a good place to start because of the influence the Greeks had on modern medicine.

2.1. The Asklepion of Hippocrates, Kos

The best site in Greece to gain a glimpse of the early history of Hippocratic medicine is on the island of Kos, close to the Turkish Mediterranean coast. This was the birthplace of Hippocrates

CHAPTER 2

(460–356 BCE), who attended one of the many Asklepions in the western Mediterranean. In Greek mythology, Apollo was the god of health, whose illegitimate son Asklepios was known for his healing power (and murdered because of it!). Healers in ancient Greece were therefore known as Asklepiads, or followers of Asklepios, and their symbol was a snake. A serpent on a rod is still a widely recognised symbol for medicine. An Asklepion was a combination of a temple and a healing place, where Asklepiads provided a combination of spiritual and health services. The ill would attend for a few days for an assessment, and then buy or make an offering to the gods that represented the diseased part of their body. This offering was called a "votive" and was often a clay model. Patients would sleep outside for a night, often after taking a prescribed medicine that was probably a sedative, so that during sleep the gods might visit, take the votive and consider healing them. Treatment options were limited, and the prognosis was up to the gods. This was really another version of "religious medicine" or supernatural healing, perhaps not too far removed from that still seen in sites such as Lourdes, and even during the recent COVID-19 pandemic.

Hippocrates followed his father into learning the healing arts. He took medicine to a new level by combining his original training with the power of careful observation of people with illnesses. As a result, he wrote a long list of *Aphorisms* – brief descriptions of symptoms and signs, generally with diagnostic and prognostic information, much of which remains accurate. After his studies and travels around most of the Mediterranean and Middle East, he settled back in Kos, converting the Asklepion there into the classical world's largest and most famous health clinic, and included in it probably Europe's first real medical school. Wealthy people travelled from far and wide to receive attention, contributing to the development of the island. Aspiring physicians would attach themselves to healers and learn from experience. The school became a powerhouse of didactic medicine, producing many textbooks based on Hippocratic observation and ethical constructs. There are so many books that it is unlikely that Hippocrates himself could have written them all, but the school had several famous physicians in the Hippocratic tradition. His greatest modern legacy is almost certainly the view of professionalism and commitment to "doing no harm". Many medical graduates recite at graduation a statement based on versions of the Hippocratic Oath.

The Asklepion was a series of buildings on three terraces in the hills four kilometres west of the town of Kos. Hippocrates believed in fresh air, clean water and healthy food, and Kos was recognised for its water supply and rich agricultural industry. It has also been at the crossroads of civilisation for over 4,000 years and has been an important trading port and cultural melting pot. The easiest way to get to the Asklepion from the town is by taxi, but for less than half the price a "mini-train" (actually a truck pulling trailers) does the journey every hour, on the hour. The entry fee includes no information on the archaeological site at all, so visitors should either purchase beforehand one of the guidebooks or book a guided tour in the language of choice.

The entire site is in ruins as a result of a large earthquake in 554 CE, after which the clinic faded under the pressure of another invasion. However, there is still much to be seen and local pamphlets provide detailed plans and images of a reconstruction based on an interpretation of the ruins. The first level included the entry halls, some patient accommodation, and probably the teaching facilities. The second level is mostly the religious buildings, with the Temple of Asklepios, Temple of Apollo and

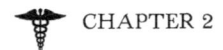

the priests' quarters. The third level has a larger temple and more patient rooms. From the top can be seen a wonderful view over the town and across the narrow waterway to Turkey. The ambience is peaceful, and the combination of peace with healthy food, water and air could be seen as a precursor to the modern health farm concept. It is easy to imagine people coming here to feel better.

The rest of Kos is well worth a visit. As a result of the invasions by just about every warlike civilisation in history (including Trojans, Spartans, Persians, Minoans, Phoenicians, Romans, Venetians, Franks, Flemish, Turks and Nazi Germany), there is a fascinating combination of architectural styles and peaceful coexistence of historic Jewish, Christian and Islamic cultures, with large churches, synagogues and mosques.

The old port fort is worth a visit, although it is relatively modern (most of the current structure dates from the fifteenth or sixteenth century), and there are ancient Roman markets, baths and theatres. Near the fort is the Hippocratic tree, allegedly the oldest and largest plane tree in the world, lovingly tended by the townsfolk as it is claimed, but cannot be proven, that Hippocrates planted it and taught students underneath it.

The island also offers several beaches, day trips to Turkey (Pergamon and Knidos are not far away) and other Greek islands, interesting old town markets, and several outdoor restaurants, so a visit does not have to be just about the history of medical education.

Further reading

2001 Summer Dream Editions. *Kos.* Stelios Kontaratos, Athens, 2001.

Chadwick, J. and Mann W.N. *The Medical Works of Hippocrates.* Blackwell Scientific Publications, Oxford, 1950.

Sigerist, H.E. *A History of Medicine. Volume II. Early Greek, Hindu and Persian Medicine*. Oxford University Press, New York, 1961.

Springer, C. "Cos and Hippocrates. A Historical Revision." *British Medical Journal*, 16 October, 1943, vol. 2, p. 492.

Location: Kos lies in the eastern Mediterranean Sea, south-east of Athens and close to Turkey.

Easiest access: The island is a 1-hour flight from Athens or a 1-hour ferry ride from Bodrum in Turkey. The Asklepion is about 22 km from the airport and 4 km from the main town of Kos.

Website: www.kos.gr/en/kos/SitePages/hippocrates.aspx

General interest to medical history:		★★★★☆	
Relevance to medical education history:		★★★★★	
Ease of access:		★★★★☆	
Tourists	X	Researchers	

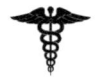

CHAPTER 3:
TURKEY

Turkey is a large and diverse nation that has always been on the junction of two continents – Europe and Asia. This is of course an oversimplification, because Turkey either now includes, formerly included, or is adjacent to the locations of several ancient, pre-European cultures. Ancient Greece at one stage included most of Turkey, just as the Ottoman Empire at one stage included Greece, most of the Middle East, part of north Africa and much of eastern and central Europe. Because of its long coastline on the Mediterranean, Caspian and Marmara Seas, there is a very long history of sea trade and movement of peoples, languages and cultures. It is no surprise then that Turkey has something to offer those with an interest in the history of medical education.

There are four sites in two Turkish cities of particular relevance to the history of medical education – one that was part of ancient Greece and provides insight into that era of medical practice and one that was the centre of the Ottoman Empire and therefore was a focus for the blending of Islamic and Christian medicine.

3.1. Bergama Asklepion

Bergama is the Turkish city that was based on the ancient Greek city of Pergamon. The ruins of that ancient city still exist and are in reasonable condition. Among the ruins is what is left

of a Greek Asklepion, similar to that found on Kos. This site is neither as impressive nor as accessible as Kos but is so close to Kos that it is possible to visit both sites within the same trip.
Location: Bergama is in south-western Turkey, close to the Mediterranean coast. Izmir is the closest city.

Easiest access: Bergama is about 2-3 hours drive north of Izmir, which is itself a 1-hour flight from Istanbul. An alternative is to take a ferry from Kos to Bodrum and travel north by car or bus.

Website: muze.gov.tr/muze-detay?SectionId=ASK01&DistId=ASK

General interest to medical history:		★★★☆☆	
Relevance to medical education history:		★★★☆☆	
Ease of access:		★★☆☆☆	
Tourists	X	Researchers	

3.2. Cerrahpasa Museum of the History of Medicine, University of Istanbul

This large, three-level museum has occupied the former medical school building from the early twentieth century. Most of the collection is about the late Ottoman Empire period (nineteenth to early twentieth centuries) and the subsequent history of the school since the establishment of the modern nation of Turkey. The latter is of less interest to international visitors, although the collection is well documented and nicely displayed, along with works of art by well-known Turkish doctors.

Displays relating to the Ottoman Empire period are more interesting, demonstrating a strong connection with military medicine, which appears to have been at the centre of professional development during that period. The medical school was at one time

CHAPTER 3

even called "The Medical School of the Ottoman Empire", as its main role was to train the military surgeons who travelled far and wide with the army that controlled the Empire. Much of the material on display concerns surgery on the battlefield, military medical uniforms and military medals awarded to battlefield surgeons. Of interest is a strong French influence in medicine during the mid-nineteenth century; France was a supporter of the Ottoman Empire at the time.

The more modern period is represented by a display of early clinical technology (huge ECG and EEG machines and sterilisation equipment) and documentation of early research activity. This section is like that found in most medical museums.

Of perhaps more interest to those with an interest in early Islamic medicine is a large collection of very intricate coloured drawings from the early Ottoman Empire period. These demonstrate heavy religious influence on life at the time and include images of medical procedures. Trephination is demonstrated, but the dominant themes are childbirth (and associated complications) and circumcision, which was clearly a big (and dangerous) step for teenage Turkish boys. Complications (bleeding, penile damage and infection) were common and it is unclear how much analgesia was available. There is also a sizeable display of circumcision instruments which might cause male observers to tremble!

One important consideration in visiting this museum is that all brochures, signs and explanation are in Turkish, so this is not an easy museum to explore without some knowledge of the Turkish language. German is more widely spoken than English and is more useful when talking with the museum staff, who want to be helpful across language barriers. Also, be aware that only the first level of the museum is usually open to the public, with the other two levels open by negotiation. The Islamic artwork is on the first level, and the other two levels house the Ottoman Empire and twentieth century collections.

TURKEY

Further reading

Ozaydin, Zuhal. "Some landmarks in the history of medicine in Istanbul (Materials, Books, Documents, Periodicals and Buildings)." *Journal of the International Society for the History of Islamic Medicine,* vol. 3. 2004, pp. 26-29.

Sari, N. "Educating the Ottoman physician." *History of Medicine Studies,* 1988; 40–64.

Location: The museum lies within the large teaching hospital complex in the old city of Istanbul, close to the southern coastline of the peninsula.

Easiest access: Istanbul airport has an extensive airline network and excellent public transport. The nearest tram stop is Yusufpasa and there are buses to the hospital, but a taxi might be the easiest transport. The museum as just inside the north entrance to the hospital campus.

Website: istanbulc.edu.tr/en/content/museums-and-exhibition-areas/cerrahpasa-museum-of-the-history-of-medicine

General interest to medical history:	★★★★☆
Relevance to medical education history:	★★★☆☆
Ease of access:	★★★☆☆
Tourists — X	*Researchers* —

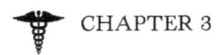
CHAPTER 3

3.3. Topkapi Palace Museum, Istanbul

The palace is a large, sprawling site on the tip of the Istanbul Peninsula, once the home of the royal family and now a national museum that contains a wide variety of treasures and historical displays. There are two sites within the complex that are of particular interest to students of medical history. The first is the medical site within the Harem, and the second is the physician's office and circumcision room in the new palace area. Clearly princes could suffer and recuperate from their circumcisions in private in a secluded and beautifully decorated tiled room! It is really only the rooms that are available to visitors and most information is in Turkish, with only very brief summaries in English. The sites do, however, convey something of the life of personal physicians to the Sultan's family – a privileged life!

Location: Within the Topkapi Palace grounds.

Easiest access: Istanbul airport has an extensive airline network and excellent public transport. The nearest tram stop is Gulhana, but it is a short walk from the two great Mosques at the Sultanahmet tram stop. The two sites are within separate sections some distance inside the main entrance.

Website: www.topkapipalace.com/

General interest to medical history:	★★☆☆☆
Relevance to medical education history:	★☆☆☆☆
Ease of access:	★★★☆☆

Tourists	X	Researchers	

3.4. Istanbul University Library

For dedicated researchers of Turkish and Islamic medical history, a range of rare manuscripts is kept at the main university library. These are not easily accessible without special access arrangements. None of the material is in any modern European language, so the company of a Turkish-speaking guide is essential, and knowledge of Latin, ancient Greek and Arabic is helpful.

Accessing the library is complex. International users must apply for access through their local Turkish Embassy and allow three months for permission to be granted.

Location: Istanbul University, Beyazit campus. This is hard to find without a guide as this is a very large, multi-campus university.

Easiest access: Istanbul airport has an extensive airline network and excellent public transport. The nearest tram stops are Üniversite and Beyazit.

Website: www.akdn.org/architecture/project/beyazit-state-library-renovation

General interest to medical history:	★☆☆☆☆	
Relevance to medical education history:	★★★☆☆	
Ease of access:	★☆☆☆☆	
Tourists	*Researchers*	X

CHAPTER 4:
ITALY

Italy is a great place for a holiday – art, contemporary design, food and wine – but also offers a number of sites relevant to history of medical education. Italy has an important place in the history of university education, because several of the developed world's first modern universities were established here, arising from cathedral schools for the clergy. The order of these sites is in approximate historical date order, but visits could be in any order.

Until about the sixth or seventh century formal medical education in Europe appears to have been available only in Greece and the Arab countries further east. In general, religious institutions were the only source of both health care and formal education. The study of medicine moved to universities during the thirteenth century.

4.1. National Historic Museum of Healthcare Art, Rome

Rome was of course the centre of the Roman Empire, which in addition to conquering much of the then known world, adopted and nurtured Greek medicine. Galen was brought to Rome to serve the political elite, and his influence on Roman medicine ensured that Greek medicine was spread and nurtured throughout the Roman Empire. Galen is famous for his anatomy text books that became an essential learning tool for many centuries, until it was realised that it was based on animal rather than human dissection. The main contribution of the post-Galenic period was the invention of surgical instruments and associated advances in surgery. Present-day Rome is an amazing place with many structures from Roman times still present, but in terms of medical education history, there is surprisingly little to see. Galen and other physicians of the time mostly cared for the wealthy, powerful classes; it is unclear just how much this affected the lives of ordinary people. Further, while the Roman Empire spread Greek medicine widely, the collapse of the Empire left little evidence of further development. In fact, the threads of medical practice do not appear for several centuries after the end of the Empire.

There are, however, some things to see. The first is the Roman ruins themselves, as they convey some of the lifestyle, culture and ambience of the Galenic period. One can imagine him attending powerful people in the magnificent buildings. There is a medical history museum at the University of Rome, but the museum was not open on several visits to Rome. It may be worth looking to see if it is open.

There is also a small medical museum within the hospital complex not far from the Vatican. Opening times are restricted so a visit requires planning. This museum is within an interesting old building set below current ground level, like much of ancient Rome. It combines a chapel, a small collection of medical art, and a small collection of surgical instruments.

Location: Presso L'Ospedale di S. Spirito, Lungotevere in Sassia 3, on the river not far from the Vatican.

Easiest access: By foot over the Ponte Vittorio Emanuale II bridge from the old city area. There are also regular buses on

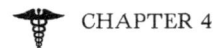
CHAPTER 4

many routes to the hospital. There is a sign inside the entrance gate off Lungotevere in Sassia, not far from the bridge.

Website: www.museiscientificiroma.eu/artesanitaria/storia.htm

General interest to medical history:		★★★☆☆	
Relevance to medical education history:		★★☆☆☆	
Ease of access:		★★☆☆☆	
Tourists	X	*Researchers*	

4.2. House of the Surgeon, Pompeii

Pompeii is one of the most famous archaeological sites in Europe and many Australians visit. I expect many will ask: what relevance does it have to the history of medical practice? Tucked away in the north-eastern tip of the site, near the Porto Ercolano, lies the House of the Surgeon. This was uncovered as part of the excavation of the site that began in the mid-eighteenth century, and so provides a glimpse into how medicine was practised in 79 CE in southern Italy. Pompeii was a relatively wealthy and powerful city-state of about 20,000 people, about 2,000 of whom perished under the volcanic debris and pyroclastic flows from nearby Mt Vesuvius. The House of the Surgeon is a relatively large complex of clinic and living rooms around a typical Roman garden. The excavation found iron and bronze surgical and obstetric implements, now housed in the Archaeological Museum in Naples. The building is on about the highest point of the city; was this accidental, related to social status, or perhaps an early manifestation of the tendency to place health facilities on high ground, surrounded by healthier air? The size is also amazing – it suggests that even 2,000 years ago some doctors were relatively wealthy.

What do we know about how medicine and surgery was practised around the time Pompeii was destroyed? First, there is no record of formal medical education in Italy at this time, so any trained doctors were most likely trained in Greece or elsewhere. Italy had once been a part of the Greek Empire, and indeed Herculaneum, less than twenty kilometres north, was a Greek city, allegedly founded by Hercules. Second, we know that many surgical procedures had been performed for centuries before this. Examples include trepanation for head injuries, amputations, removal of near-term infants after the mother's death (remembered as Caesarean sections), fracture reduction with traction devices and suturing of wounds. Most of the development in surgical practice came from dealing with trauma, particularly that arising from wars. Surgical outcomes were limited by poor anaesthesia and inability to manage bleeding, although hashish, opium and mandragora root (mixed with wine) were used for analgesia, and wound cauterisation was known.

Location: Just south of Naples.

Easiest access: By car or train (local Circumvesuviana line) from Naples (30 minutes), and Rome (3.5 hours). Ferries run regular services along the scenic coast from Sorrento and the Amalfi coast to Torre Annunziata.

Website: www.pompeionline.net/en/archaeological-park-of-pompeii/houses-of-pompeii

General interest to medical history:		★☆☆☆☆
Relevance to medical education history:		★☆☆☆☆
Ease of access:		★★★★☆
Tourists	X	*Researchers*

4.3. Virtual Museum of Salerno's Medical School

Salerno is a bit off the normal tourist itinerary but is easily accessible for those who want to travel to places where English is less often understood, ordinary Italian life is more visible, and prices are lower. This is the site of possibly the first medical school in modern Europe, established in about the sixth or seventh century by Greek graduates of the Alexandria school The choice of Salerno probably related to its location in the "Greek" part of Italy and perhaps its "healthy" Mediterranean climate. Because of its location – at the crossroads of several cultures and warring empires – its practitioners were influenced by a combination of Arab, Jewish, Greek, Roman and African health concepts to form the basis of the new, "Latin" medical school tradition. Unlike the later European medical schools, it was not formally affiliated with either the church or a university. Perhaps because of its independence, women were admitted as both students and teachers, and a book on diseases of women was produced.[1,2] Because the early days of the Salerno school are poorly documented, there is some uncertainty about the period that has provoked mythical and romantic reconstructions of what may well have been very pragmatic decisions.[3]

The school's most influential period was from around 1070 to the late thirteenth century. Its main strengths were in internal medicine, wound management (particularly skull wounds) and the use of uroscopy (diagnosis based on the urine's colour, concentration and smell, and the presence of foam, mucous or blood). One famous physician was Constantine the African, who is credited with bringing Arab medicine into modern European life. Constantine spent thirty-nine years learning his trade by wandering across Arabia to India and back via Ethiopia and Carthage. He later settled in Monte Cassino, not far from Salerno, converted to Christianity, became a monk, and died in 1087. He was only one of many wandering physicians and philosophers who helped to establish Salerno as a centre of medical learning.

Notable patients enhanced the school's reputation. For example, local practitioners saved the life of the Norman conqueror Robert Guiscard, who was seriously ill with infected wounds from the Crusades.[1] In return, Robert supported the school and it became the pre-eminent medical school of its time, with its graduates recognised widely. Uroscopy was popular for many centuries as it linked health to the spiritual world of the time. Because of the Norman link, some of the Salerno textbooks were translated and imported to other lands, including England.

The Salerno school was a pioneer in medical education because it developed a curriculum that included philosophy and logic – the Salernitan approach.[3] Entering students had to have completed three years of preparatory studies, and then embarked on a five-year theoretical course, followed by one year of supervised practice. Staff produced many classic textbooks of the day, both originals and Latin translations of many of the works of Galen and Hippocrates. *The Regimen Sanitas Salernitum*, the most famous, is a rhyming didactic poem, in Latin, of more than 300 verses, covering a wide range of health problems, diagnoses and treatments.[4] This school is also said to be the first to use examinations – entirely *viva voce* (oral) – with set standards of knowledge. Physicians had to pass these examinations before practising and had to abide by a code of conduct that, for example, forbade partnerships with apothecaries. Further, teachers had to be qualified physicians.

Anatomy and surgery were not strengths of the school as human dissection was not permitted (that came later), although pigs were dissected and a surgeon – Roger (Rogerius) of Salerno – wrote one of the definitive surgical textbooks of the era. Another example of pioneering is the twelfth century writing about the use of early anaesthesia techniques. Yet another is the expansion of knowledge about pharmacy and medicines, with a book on prescriptions written by Nicolai around the same time.

After Roger moved on, the impetus for developing medical practice declined, although some form of medical school is said to have survived until the early nineteenth century. The lack of formal university and church affiliation probably contributed to its gradual fading, as did several earthquakes – Salerno is one of the most-often destroyed Italian cities because it lies on an earthquake fault. The final straw appears to have been conquest by Napoleon's army in 1811.

As a result of the repeated destruction of the town, which was again badly damaged in World War II, little remains to indicate the location, size and scope of this important episode in history. Salerno is still worth a visit, however, just to take in the ambience of the healthy southern Italian coastline and to observe the Moorish influence on architecture in the surrounding towns. There is a "virtual museum" of the medical school the Church of San Gregorio and an interesting archaeology museum that covers remains of earlier Salerno habitation from around the first century CE.

References

1. Puschmann, T. A. and Hare, E.H. *History of Medical Education.* [Translated and edited by E.H. Hare] Facsimile of 1891 ed. Hafner, New York 1966.

2. Singer, C. and Singer, D. "The origin of the medical school of Salerno, the first University. An attempted reconstruction." In *Essays on the History of Medicine presented to Karl Sudhoff on the occasion of his seventieth birthday November 26, 1923.* Eds: Singer C. and Sigerist H.E., Oxford University Press, London, 1924.

3. Kristeller P. The school of Salerno: its development and its contribution to the history of learning. Bulletin of the History of Medicine, 1945; 17: 138-194. 4. Guthrie, D. *A History of Medicine*. Thomas Nelson & Sons, London, 1945. Reprinted 1960.

4. Parente, P.P. *The Regimen of Health of The Medical School of Salerno*. Vantage Press, New York, 1967.

Location: Just south of the Amalfi coast. Virtual Museum of Salerno's Medical School, Chiesa di San Gregorio, via dei Mercanti 74, Salerno; Archaeological Museum, via San Benedetto, 28 Complesso Abbaziale San Benedetto.

Easiest access: By car or train from Naples (1 hour) and Rome (4 hours). Ferries also run services along the scenic coast from Sorrento and the Amalfi coast.

Websites: www.livesalerno.com/virtual-museum-of-salerno-s-medical-school; www.livesalerno.com/provincial-archaeological-museum

General interest to medical history:		★★☆☆☆
Relevance to medical education history:		★★★☆☆
Ease of access:		★☆☆☆☆
Tourists	X	Researchers

4.4. Anatomical Theatre, University of Padova

Padova (Padua) is a small university city, similar in concept to Oxford, credited with being the site of the first formal medical school in modern Europe (Salerno has nobody left to argue against that!) within Europe's second oldest university. It is also where medical education took a major leap forward and into the unknown through the introduction of anatomy teaching based on then-illegal human dissection. It has arguably the most impressive example of an anatomy demonstration theatre in the world. The city of 250,000 people is about thirty minutes by fast train inland from Venice. The university has 63,000 students, so higher education is the main business. A ten-minute walk from the train station brings you to the ancient walled city and two blocks south on via 8 Febbraio is the original University of Padova building that contains the first medical school facilities.

In 1222 the university took over an old tavern – The Ox – opposite the Palace of Justice in the centre of Padova. Medicine was part of the arts faculty until 1319, when it became a separate school. In 1543 a Belgian anatomist, Andreas Vesalius, one of the pioneers of human dissection, moved to Padova and commenced dissection of human cadavers. This was not legal, so was done clandestinely. Cadavers of Christians could not be used because of the dominant view at the time that the body must be complete for the soul to travel to heaven. To circumvent this strict law in a Christian state the school obtained the bodies of Jewish criminals who had been convicted and hanged in the Palace of Justice just over the road. There was a substantial Jewish enclave living in Padova at the time and either their religion locally did not oppose dissection (this was a contentious issue) or a blind eye was turned by the authorities, so long as discretion was maintained. Hence the bodies would be secretly brought in under cover of darkness to a small preparation room adjacent to a specially designed "secret" anatomy demonstration theatre.

The anatomy suite is upstairs and has an oval shape that is hidden within the square external contours of the building. It packs six narrow tiers of standing room for up to 300 people into about forty feet of vertical space under a large domed ceiling. The timber construction provides high rails on each tier designed so that students who fainted (usually from the smell of decomposing bodies) could not fall into the circle and land on the cadaver or teacher. A cadaver would be placed on a marble slab that could be raised into the demonstration table from a passage connected to the preparation room. Should the authorities come looking for an illegal dissection, the body could be moved to a trolley and pushed out through the corridor and dumped into the stream below, removing the evidence!

Vesalius did not stay in Padova long, as he established a reputation that made him famous and in demand. He wrote the first anatomy text based on human anatomy – up till then Galen's anatomy treatise was the definitive text, but it was probably based on primate dissection and therefore not completely accurate for humans. Galen's work was functionally accurate, and Vesalius' criticism of the revered Galen made him controversial. He later returned to France to be personal physician to Charles V.

Next to the demonstration theatre is the Medical Salon, a large room where students sat on benches against walls and teaching staff sat in ornate leather armchairs around a central table. From here they would provide didactic teaching and also conduct annual examinations, which were entirely by viva voce in the Salerno tradition. The walls of the Salon are full of wonderful artworks, mostly portraits of early teachers, including Eustachio (as in tubes) and Morgagni (as in crypts of), and medical diagrams. The

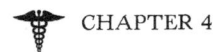

corridors and halls of the whole complex are decorated with the family crests of early graduates, but there has been no room for more of these for a couple of centuries.

The tradition of viva examinations is still strong in Padova, as is a rather loud public graduation ceremony. Such ceremonies still take place all year round and during a visit you may hear groups singing a song that ends in "oom-pa-pa" as hats are thrown high into the air and photos are taken.

Location: Padova, Northern Italy

Easiest access: By car or train (40 minutes from Venice).

Website: www.unipd.it/en/palazzo-bo-and-anatomical-theatre

General interest to medical history:		★★☆☆☆	
Relevance to medical education history:		★★★★★	
Ease of access:		★★★★☆	
Tourists	X	*Researchers*	

4.5. Anatomical Theatre, University of Bologna

Bologna is a large city of one million people and has its own cuisine and a history of freethinking and radical politics. It is worth a visit just for the eating and shopping but is also the site of the first medical school in the modern western world that offered a recognised university degree in medicine, a privilege bestowed in 1268 by Pope Clement IV. Bologna had developed as a university that trained the religious, and like most early European universities, had just two faculties – Law and Arts. The former primarily taught canon and civil law, while the latter included philosophy, mathematics, physics, the natural sciences and, from the thirteenth century, medicine. Early medical education included instruction in astrology, herbs and what could loosely be called anatomy and physiology, although not as we know it today. Anatomy teaching, where present, was initially based on dissection of animals, because Church law forbade human dissection on the grounds that the entire body had to be buried in order for the soul to travel to heaven. European medical education grew more powerful and here in Bologna became a separate university discipline during the fourteenth century. The medical school is credited with the development of the two-part medical training, with a *studium* (theoretical training) followed by a *practicum* (clinical experience). Several small museums offer a fascinating insight into early medical education here.

Initially anatomy teaching was based on animal dissection, as elsewhere, but after the successful introduction of human dissection in Padova, Bologna built its own Teatro Anatomica within the main university building. This building is located in via dell'Archiginnasio, inside the Museo Civico Archeologico, close to the old centre of the city and across the road from the Basilica di San Petronio, a popular tourist haunt. This building consolidated the previously scattered schools that made up the university's two disciplines – law and the arts. The anatomy demonstration theatre was built in 1637 on the second level at the rear of the courtyard, close to the Ospedale della Morte (hospital of death). By this time anatomy dissection was more accepted and done more openly. The theatre design was more spacious than that in Padova, built as a rectangle with three tiers of timber-seated benches around the central marble slab dissection table. The tiers are not steep, and the view afforded to those seated in the benches would not be as good as in the original Padova design. On the other hand, accessibility and ventilation are much improved, reflecting the relaxation of

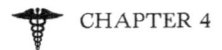CHAPTER 4

the law at the time. The walls and ceilings are decorated ornately with statues of famous anatomists and of Apollo. The theatre was rebuilt after heavy bombing raid damage in 1944.

Location: Piazza Galvani 1, 40124, Bologna, northern Italy.

Easiest access: Reach Bologna by car or train from Rome (2 hours), Florence (1 hour) or Venice (2 hours); the nearest bus stop is Piazza Maggiore.

Website: www.archiginnasio.it/visit.htm

4.6. Museum of Palazzo Poggi, Bologna University

Two fascinating collections are housed within the Museo Università in Palazzo Poggi, the central university museum. The first is the anatomy collection, which was moved only recently from the anatomy department (some guidebooks provide the wrong address). Established in 1742 by Pope Benedict XIV, this collection consists of mostly waxwork models of various body parts and of the creators of much of the collection – Dr and Signora Manzoni. Dr Manzoni was an anatomy teacher and his wife the model maker. The models were created at a time when human dissection could play only a limited role because specimens could not be kept long. There are several models of the musculoskeletal system (limbs with bones, muscles, nerves and vessels), the abdomen, the chest, the face, the brain, the larynx and others depicting trauma. The models are to scale and are amazingly realistic, being much more like what surgeons see than preserved specimens. Indeed, they continued to be used in teaching until the early 1900s.

The second collection is a collection of models depicting normal and abnormal obstetric practices, established by Dr Giovanni Galli, a teacher of midwives and surgeons. The models are of stages of fetal and uterine development, every possible presentation in labour and complications and their management. The models are to scale, made of clay, coloured appropriately and also incredibly realistic, conveying a three-dimensional image far better than any drawing. I would have benefited from seeing these models before practising rural obstetrics! Also included are a set of obstetric implements and an operative delivery table of the era. The collection was donated to the university in 1757 by the Vatican. Both collections are open to the public seven days a week during summer months. If your Italian is good enough, more information can be obtained by calling the museum.

Location: via Zamboni 33, 40126 Bologna.

Easiest access: The nearest bus stop is Porta San Donato.

Website: sma.unibo.it/en/the-university-museum-network/luigi-cattaneo-anatomical-wax-collection/luigi-cattaneo-anatomical-wax-collection

General interest to medical history:		★★★★☆
Relevance to medical education history:		★★★★★
Ease of access:		★★★★☆
Tourists	X	Researchers

4.7. La Specola, National History Museum, University of Florence

Florence has so many interesting museums that celebrate the fantastic era of Renaissance art and sculpture, but there are other treasures too. Within the art museums can be found paintings by two of the most famous artists with an interest in human anatomy – Leonardo da Vinci and Michelangelo. About halfway to Pisa is

CHAPTER 4

the town of Vinci, Leonardo's hometown, where there are several museums that honour the local hero and exhibit collections relevant to both his art and his scientific inventions. There are good rail and bus connections from both Florence and Pisa.

A less well-known fact is that Florence also made a major contribution to medical education by being home to a blend of art and science. In the Oltarno section of Florence, just south of the Ponte Vecchio, is a museum called La Specola. Part of the Università degli studi Firenze, this is a must for those interested in medical history as it houses a fine collection of life-sized wax models of human anatomy that were used as teaching aids. Getting to the anatomy collection requires navigation through a majority of the thirty-four rooms that contain stuffed real animals or life-sized models of them. There are so many animals that this seems to be the museum equivalent of Noah's Ark, except that there is usually only one of each. The collection predates the modern preference for viewing animals in wildlife parks and breeding endangered species, but it contains some now extinct species.

If the normal path is followed by museum visitors, the last few rooms include human anatomy drawings and models made at the Florence school of wax modelling. This was not the first place to construct such detailed, coloured models – that credit goes to Bologna, where it was pioneered by Gaetamo Giulio Zumbo – but it may have been the first of the large, comprehensive collections; several master modellers were trained here. The original use of the models was to aid teaching, as there were not enough cadavers available for dissection-based teaching. The collection was established in the late eighteenth century (most models are labelled as being made between 1775 and 1791), although some were made as late as about 1830, and survived World War II by being hidden. The master wax modellers at Florence were Ferreni,

Susini, Matteucci and Valvani, although they had several helpers. The models were based on some of the original anatomical drawings by Eustacchio and Albinus, although the modellers also had access to specimens dissected within the school. The walls are covered with coloured drawings that guided the modellers. This is the original, largest and most famous collection, from which many copies were made. These copies are now in several other collections, the largest of them in Austria at the Josephinum collection (see Austria 1). They can also be seen in other museums elsewhere in Italy, in Montpellier (see France 1), Leiden in the Netherlands (see Netherlands 1) and even in the Wellcome Galleries at the Science Museum in London (see England 1).

The models cover just about everything, but for me the most interesting are the models that display the lymphatic and vascular systems. The detail is fine-grained and arguably better than the more recent plastinated models. There is also a large collection relevant to obstetrics. In many ways the collection is a more realistic teaching aid as the colours are more lifelike than real body parts preserved in formalin.

Easiest access: Via Romana 17, 5125 Florence. This is an easy walk in central Florence, just south of the Ponte Vecchio and just past the Palazzo Pitti. The museum is on the second floor, an old building with about sixty steps! The nearest airports are Florence and Pisa, but Rome is only about 2 hours away by train.

Website: www.msn.unifi.it/vp-387-la-specola.html?newlang=eng

General interest to medical history:		★★☆☆☆	
Relevance to medical education history:		★★★☆☆	
Ease of access:		★★★★☆	
Tourists	X	*Researchers*	

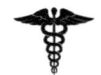

CHAPTER 5:
SPAIN

Around about the time that Salerno was developing as a Mediterranean cultural melting pot, a similar development was occurring in southern Spain. The Roman Empire had developed a strong province in Baetica, now Andalusia. This area had a combination of productive olive groves and good port access for trade with north Africa, Italy, Greece, Syria and Egypt. Hence the region had people of many cultures living together. As the Roman Empire waned, with Italian influence retracting to central and northern Italy, the influence of other cultures increased. Moorish culture was literally just across the narrow opening of the Mediterranean Sea, and Islamic leaders moved in with a series of violent invasions, establishing a dominance that would last for about three centuries, as the centre of the western caliphate. Jewish culture was also strong, and the Christian kings returned later to establish and cement Christianity as the dominant religion, at times also using harsh measures to rid the country of other religions. However, while these three religions battled for dominance, the province was for about three centuries a thriving multicultural centre that produced great thinkers and philosophers from all three religions. Because at the time medicine was very closely related to philosophy, the practice of medicine flourished, breaking new ground, both in philosophical and pharmaceutical developments. The influence of Andalusia is all the more remarkable for its multi-faith contributions over a considerable period of time.

Four of the greatest early medical philosophers became prominent in the Andalusian region. The first three were Arab Muslims. The first was Albucasis (936–1013), who wrote a complete account of medicine and surgery. The second was Avenzoar (1091–1162), who discovered the tick mite and wrote a textbook based on careful observation of clinical cases. The third was his student, Averroes, also known as Ibn Rushd (1126–1198), who wrote a textbook before being imprisoned for having ideas that were too freethinking. The thinking of these three, as well as most in the western caliphate, was philosophically different from that of Avicenna in the east.[1]

The fourth was the Jew Maimonides, also known as Rambam (1135–1204), who is remembered as a jurist, philosopher, physician and religious adviser. The son of a judge, he received a very broad education and developed an early interest in Aristotle's work, which he re-interpreted in Jewish religious thinking. Amidst one of the more turbulent periods of Islamic invasion, the family moved several times within Spain, before moving to north Africa and then to Palestine in 1167. Soon after they moved to Egypt, which had earlier been the centre of Arab medicine. Maimonides returned to Cordoba in 1173, where he remained for many years as a medical practitioner. Islam was more tolerant of Judaism than Christianity, and so Jews could live in relative safety under all except the most extreme Islamic rulers. Here he wrote several tracts that were used by European medical schools until the age of scientific rationalism, including a commentary on the work of Galen and a pharmacopoeia.[2,3] He also wrote an oath for graduating physicians that has been used as an alternative to the various interpretations of the Hippocratic Oath. Despite being a native Hebrew speaker, he wrote in Arabic. Like his mentor Averroes, he ran into difficulties because of his unusual views on religious philosophy; both were criticised for their difficulty reconciling reason and logic with unswerving belief in God.[4]

5.1. Old Quarter, Cordoba

Sadly, nothing specific to medical practice survives from the tenth to twelfth centuries, but Cordoba is a fascinating place, rich in cultural and religious heritage. At its peak the city is said to have had a population of 250,000, with many mosques and fine buildings and a thriving, tolerant regime that was inclusive of the different cultures. The area to visit is the old quarter, surrounding the large central mosque and cathedral complex by the river and opposite the Roman bridge. The mosque (known locally as the Mezquita) is a most unusual complex that began as a mosque, but later had a cathedral built within it. This is a very old structure, dating in parts from 785, and has several additions and re-builds according to the dominant culture and religion of the time. It consists of a large square building that is half garden courtyard and half covered hall; this hall is around the size of two football (soccer) fields. Inside the hall is much more similar to other mosques, with large open spaces around over 800 columns that support the roof. The arches, the doors and the windows appear to be heavily influenced by Islamic architecture, but in the centre is a classical Christian section that would not be out of place in any other cathedral.[5]

It is believed that somewhere here was a medical school that built on the work of the Arab physicians and Maimonides. The Mezquita is more-or-less surrounded by a "Jewish quarter" that contains markets and a synagogue built in 1315 in Calle Judios, close to Maimonides Place.

Nothing remains of the school, and its location is not even known, although some observers believe that it may have been either in, or very close to, the Mezquita. However, it is worthwhile wandering around the old city, absorbing the atmosphere. With its very narrow streets (room for a tiny car or two to three pedestrians at a time, but not both), numerous craft markets and fortune-tellers, this is a fascinating journey through the past. One place worth visiting is the Archaeological Museum, on Plaza de Jeronimo Paez 7, north-east of the Mezquita. While it has nothing relevant to medical practice, it contains artefacts and displays relevant to the Visigoths, Romans, Muslims, Jews and Christians that all lived here and left behind evidence of how they lived, often building on and adapting contributions from previous civilisations. There are also several small museums that house collections relating to the blending of art, craft and musical traditions.

References

1. Ead, Hamed A. Averroes as a Physician. www.levity.com/alchemy/islam21.html

2. Shapiro, John. *The Jewish 100. A Rating of the Most Influential Jews of All Time.* Citadel Press, New York, 1994.

3. Davidson, H.A. *Moses Maimonides. The Man and His Works.* Oxford University Press, New York, 2004.

4. Puschmann T. and Hare, E.H. *A History of Medical Education.* [Translated and edited by E.H. Hare] Facsimile of 1891 ed., Hafner, New York, 1966.

5. *Cordoba Guidebook.* Otermin Ediciones S.C.

Location: The city of Cordoba is about 200 km east-north-east from Seville, in southern Spain. The old city is along the northern riverbank.

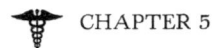

Easiest access: The nearest airport is at Seville. Express trains (40 mins travel time) and buses (about 1 hour) depart regularly from the Sant Justia Station on Ave Kansas City. Trains also connect to Madrid (1 hour 45 minutes).

Website: mezquita-catedraldecordoba.es/en/; www.museosdeandalucia.es/web/museoarqueologicodecordoba

General interest to medical history:	★☆☆☆☆
Relevance to medical education history:	★★★★☆
Ease of access:	★★☆☆☆
Tourists X	*Researchers*

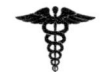

CHAPTER 6:
FRANCE

Visitors to Paris will note the pride with which Parisians speak of their cultural integrity, language and history, claiming to be the dominant European cultural influence of the last millennium. Protected during wars, Paris offers fashion, literature, theatre, food and wine.

In northern Europe, France was the early leader in medical education. Medical schools were established in the twelfth and thirteenth centuries in Montpellier, Toulouse and Paris. Montpellier claims to be the second oldest in Europe (after Salerno) and is recognised for its contribution to developments in both theory and practice. The early Paris schools were regarded as more "vocational" schools that focused on practical training and were dominated by the professions. Medical education in Britain and northern Europe developed similarly under Parisian influences. French medical researchers became world leaders by the seventeenth and eighteenth centuries, and Paris was the centre of medical specialisation, based on advances in clinical pathology during the eighteenth and nineteenth centuries. Here narrow specialisation became well accepted early and even dominated practice within a few decades. Strangely, French medical education did not follow its British cousin into clinical education but remained largely didactic and theoretical until very recently.

Medical students would have to first obtain a degree from the medical school and then apply for clinical training in unrelated, non-academic hospitals, but many failed to achieve this and so were unable to practise medicine. This strong separation between studium and practicum persisted for centuries, much later than elsewhere in Europe. Following student unrest, the system was reformed in 1968, with the by then huge, single Paris medical school split into thirteen smaller medical schools, each attached to a teaching hospital, and courses were changed to include clinical training prior to graduation.

Because Paris went on to become the dominant French city, it contains the largest number of relevant historical sites. Most are located near the Latin Quarter, perhaps the most convenient place to stay for walking to them, as here one is literally surrounded by Parisian medical school facilities. However, Paris has an efficient and easily navigable public transport system for those staying elsewhere. Visitors will get more out of the visits if they speak French, as not many places offer complete English translations to explain their collections.

Further reading

Puschmann, T. and Hare, E.H. *A History of Medical Education.* [Translated and edited by E.H. Hare] Facsimile of 1891 ed. Hafner, New York 1966.

Guthrie, D. *A History of Medicine.* Thomas Nelson and Sons, London, 1945. Reprinted 1960.

Weisz, G. *Divide and Conquer: A comparative history of medical specialisation.* Oxford University Press, New York, 2005.

6.1. Montpellier Medical School

Close to the French Mediterranean coast, this modern multicultural city is the site of France's first medical school. Its origins were probably earlier, but records show it was established in about 1135 as an independent school, similar to that in Salerno. It was founded around a health resort that attracted both patients and physicians. Unlike Salerno it was taken over by Pope Honorius III in 1220, recognised as a university and maintained. This support came at a price, because only Christians were deemed to be desirable as students and teachers.

Montpellier is another university city, with about a quarter of the population enrolled at a university, and most people on the streets seem to be under twenty-five. The old city centre is mostly pedestrian access, with narrow cobbled streets, numerous coffee shops and an efficient bus and tram city circle system. Its weather and ambience are definitely more Mediterranean than continental.

The history is long and there are some fascinating sites to visit apart from the archaeology and regional history museums, although they are not well identified. The real jewel is in the medical school in rue de l'École de Médecine, located within the pedestrianised medieval city centre. The building, originally a Benedictine Monastery and then the Bishop's Palace, was given to the medical faculty in 1794. In parts it is about 600 years old; over succeeding centuries it has suffered destruction during religious wars then been rebuilt and added to. It is worth exploration, although it is a functioning medical school and is full of offices, seminar rooms, staff and students. It is connected to the old cathedral of Saint Pierre, evidence of the early close relationship with the Church. Here too is proof of the traditional relationships between medical education, art and literature, with adjacent

CHAPTER 6

collections of art, historical manuscripts and anatomy specimens. The anatomy museum was closed for renovation for several years but has reopened, displaying some specimens from a collection in Paris that has closed. The art collection, Le Musée Atger, is hidden behind the current undergraduate library that when I was there was packed with first-year medical students studying for an exam. The museum houses a collection of 500 drawings and paintings donated in the early nineteenth century by a local benefactor. Many are drawings of the human body, dating from the sixteenth to eighteenth centuries, highlighting the connection between art and medicine. Some famous artists are represented, including Carravaggio, Ruebens, Van Dyck and Fragonard, so a visit is well worth the trouble.

La Bibliothèque (the old library) is the real highlight. Tucked away down a secluded corridor is a small room that contains replicas of many of the classic medical texts from the eighth to nineteenth centuries. The complete collections of Hippocrates, Galen and others are there to read, so long as you can read Latin. There are also many old medical dictionaries and pharmacopoeias and complete encyclopedias of botany, surgery and medicine from the last 200 years, in both Latin and French. Even more amazing is the collection of original manuscripts, which are less accessible. Here are kept copies of the original 1545 Andreas Vesalius anatomy treatise (the first based on human anatomy), a 1533 translation of Galen, and de Chauliac's pioneering textbook of surgery, written in 1363 but not printed until 1498. The anatomical drawings are as accurate as those in the modern textbooks being used by the students in the next room. Vesalius's drawings of dissected corpses in erect poses are amazing, if not a little spooky. These are priceless documents that deserve reverence!

This is not an easy site to visit without some capacity to speak French and read Latin, but the library staff members were very helpful and appreciative of the interest shown by someone from so far away. The library at least is probably mainly for those with a serious academic interest in medical history.

Location: Montpellier.

Easiest access: A 10-minute walk from Montpellier railway station, which is 5 hours by TGV from Paris and 1 hour from Marseilles.

Website: www.umontpellier.fr/patrimoine/musees/musee-danatomie; www.med.univ-montp1.fr/

General interest to medical history:		★☆☆☆☆	
Relevance to medical education history:		★★★★★	
Ease of access:		★★★★☆	
Tourists	X	*Researchers*	X

6.2. Museum of the History of Medicine, Paris

This is the best-maintained medical museum in Paris and is probably the best place to commence the Paris itinerary. It is a more general museum and its main strength is a sequence of exhibits that summarise the development of medical practice in France through time. This begins with instruments used by the ancient Gauls to conduct cataract extractions – something not mentioned in Asterix comics – and goes through to the early twentieth century. There is something to see from every era, but highlights include the depiction of the strong French contributions to neurology in the seventeenth and eighteenth centuries and urology in the nineteenth century. Famous researchers such as Dupuytren (as in contracture), Charcot (as in joint) and Pasteur have some floor space, but the main focus is on the clinical side, particularly the development of surgery and its specialties. An interesting feature is a collection of over fifty glass and wax model eyeballs, depicting in three dimensions every conceivable ocular pathology – much more real and satisfying than the colour photographs we usually rely on. I was also surprised to see how advanced endoscopy was in France more than a century ago. The museum includes paintings and statues depicting famous figures and events relevant to the themes of the display.

The building itself is worth walking around, although being a functioning medical school of the Université de Paris restricts access. This was part of the former single Paris medical school, France's second medical school, established in 1270. While not the original building, it is about 200 years old and has wide corridors, grand staircases, large lecture halls and great artwork, including sculptures and paintings. Medical schools like this are no longer built! A quick look at noticeboards indicates that each medical school year cohort has seven to eight hundred students, large by any standards. Studying and teaching in such large organisations must be challenging.

Location: School of Medicine, 12 rue de l'École de Médecine, 75006, Paris (6^E).

Easiest access: Odeon Metro station (Line 4 and 10).

Website: www.atlasobscura.com/places/museum-of-the-history-of-medicine

General interest to medical history:	★★★★☆
Relevance to medical education history:	★☆☆☆☆
Ease of access:	★★★★☆
Tourists X	*Researchers*

6.3. Museum of Public Assistance –Paris Hospitals

This museum tells the story of how Paris's first general hospital developed in the twelfth and thirteenth centuries on the Île de la Cité in central Paris, just across from Notre Dame. The original site was where the current Hôtel Dieu (general hospital) is located, but this was destroyed by fire in the 1840s and rebuilt as a more modern hospital. The museum lies across the river on Quai de la Tournelle, in Hôtel Miramion, and is said to have a similar physical structure to the original hospital, with high ceilings and the usual large, open, multi-bed wards.

The story is similar to elsewhere in Europe. The people in greatest need were the poor and the destitute, adjectives that described much of the city's population. The Church took on the role in caring for the poor, so the hospital began as an extension to church facilities, with nuns and priests providing all the care, mostly tending to the dying. There were relatively few doctors at the time; until the fourteenth century most medical students were in religious orders and the training was provided by the Church-run universities, including the new Paris medical school at the Sorbonne.

Most doctors worked privately on contracts with towns, wealthy families or royalty, but as medical ethics developed, some donated their time to work for the poor. Also, early medical teachers realised that hospitals were a source of learning, because

CHAPTER 6

of the considerable amount of pathology on view. Initially doctors donated some of their time as a religious commitment, but the access this brought to patients with interesting pathology resulted in many becoming famous clinicians. The evolution of modern nursing practice from religious orders is depicted in the museum. Over the centuries the hospital developed into one of the city's main central hospitals, although because of the separation of medical schools and hospitals, it emerged rather late as a formal teaching hospital.

The museum includes furniture, equipment and paintings from the original hospital, in surroundings that are said to be similar to the original hotel. I found the most interesting exhibit was an early twentieth century ECG machine. It was so large that it could not fit into the back of the average estate wagon, and its tangle of wires and solenoids makes more obvious the electro-physiological basis of the investigation.

This museum closed in 2012 but may reopen, so it is included. Please check the current status.

Location: 47 Quai de la Tournelle, 75005, Paris (5^E).

Easiest access: Saint-Michel Metro Station (Line 4), or across the bridge from Notre Dame on the southern side of the Seine.

General interest to medical history:		★★★☆☆
Relevance to medical education history:		★★☆☆☆
Ease of access:		★★★★☆
Tourists	X	*Researchers*

6.4. Anatomy Theatre, Paris

This site has no supporting information but can be found in the Latin Quarter by walking along the rue de la Bûcherie, away from the narrow streets of restaurants near St Michels Square, very close to the Seine and across the bridge adjacent to Notre Dame. Much of this area used to be part of the University of Paris medical school but was sold as the university expanded and consolidated. This building is the original seventeenth century anatomy demonstration theatre used by the medical school to teach anatomy. While it is not as large or as grand as the Padova theatre in Italy, it is still an attractive, approximately twenty-metre diameter, circular, stone building with a high dome. Entry is via the ground floor, where dissections took place. The seats around where the dissecting table sat have been removed and the chamber is empty. Looking upwards, an upper gallery is visible, as is a mid-level half-terrace, both for observing proceedings below.

The building is now part of a private business that occupies the adjacent building complex. When I walked in and asked if I could see inside the dome, I was given a brief tour. Access is not guaranteed but is worth asking for.

Location: Corner of rue de la Bûcherie and rue de l'Hôtel Colbert, 75005, Paris (5^E).

Easiest access: Saint-Michel Metro station (Line 4).

General interest to medical history:		★☆☆☆☆
Relevance to medical education history:		★★★☆☆
Ease of access:		★★★☆☆
Tourists	X	*Researchers*

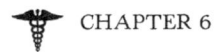

6.5. Delmas-Orfila-Rouvière Anatomy Museum, Paris

This museum houses one of the world's largest collections of normal anatomy specimens. It is located in another of Paris's now separated medical schools but is only a ten-minute walk from the medical school that houses the Musée d'Histoire. It is another large medical school with large class sizes and grand buildings that are not very old by Parisian standards.

Despite arranging to visit Paris six times at different times of the year, I have not yet managed to get inside the doors of this museum, even with a French-speaking colleague making the contact. It appears the museum is not keen on having external visitors and it is said to be closed permanently. No manner of pleading and explaining the purpose made any difference. The most plausible explanation is that most of the collection does not have clear provenance, raising serious ethical concerns but public displays of human remains gathered without consent. Some specimens are on display at the medical school at the University of Montpelier.

I have included this museum in case it re-appears or specimens are included in other local museums. Visitors to Paris are advised to check on its status, but not to be too disappointed if it does not work out.

Location: School of Medicine, 45 rue des Saints-Pères, 75006, Paris (6^E).

Easiest access: Saint-Germain des Prés Metro station (Line 4).

General interest to medical history:		★★☆☆☆	
Relevance to medical education history:		★★☆☆☆	
Ease of access:		★☆☆☆☆	
Tourists	X	Researchers	

6.6. Dupuytren Museum, Paris

This is a spectacular collection of pathological anatomy specimens and models collected mostly from the seventeenth century onwards. The main contributor was the famous surgeon Professor Dupuytren, obstetrician to Napoleon's wife. Dupuytren began as a non-clinical pathologist, as did most of France's famous medical researchers, but later became a clinical professor specialising in neurology. This museum contains an amazing array of pathology specimens of conditions that most current doctors and medical students will never see. This is why such collections can be valuable in medical education, particularly when collecting specimens is now so difficult. There are many examples of anencephaly, tuberculosis in the spine, syphilis in skulls, typhoid in the bowel and congenital abnormalities. The brain that helped Paul Broca explain aphasia and specimens from Jean-Martin Charcot are also highlights. The diagnostic content is testimony to the major public health challenges of the seventeenth, eighteenth and nineteenth centuries – very few specimens of cancer can be found here.

For me, the highlight is the collection of wax and plaster-cast models that were used for teaching. These were painstakingly modelled on real patients by wax craftsmen, who at the time were essential contributors to medical education. Few are left now, and rumour has it that in Paris their craft was saved by Madame Tussaud's wax museum. I think these are much more useful as teaching aides than pictures and pathology specimens in formalin. There is also a huge collection of original neuroanatomical glass histology slides used to describe many now famous neurological conditions, but perhaps they are of interest only to visiting neuropathologists!

CHAPTER 6

This collection is becoming harder to see as it is no longer in regular use and competition for space and resources in a growing university mean that it is hard to fund its maintenance. A lack of provenance of many specimens is a likely challenge. When I visited it was is being run by volunteers and it has since closed to the public, perhaps permanently. The collection is accessible only to researchers, medical practitioners and students, by prior arrangement. Please make contact in advance with the Sorbonne University for current information.

Location: School of Medicine, 15 rue de l'École de Médecine, 75006, Paris (6^E).

Easiest access: Odeon Metro station (lines 4 and 10).

Website: https://www.sorbonne-universite.fr/en/culture-and-outreach/noteworthy-places-collections-and-bequests/outstanding-collections-and

General interest to medical history:	★★☆☆☆
Relevance to medical education history:	★★☆☆☆
Ease of access:	★☆☆☆☆
Tourists	*Researchers* X

6.7. Paris Medical School Library

Located in the same building as the Musée d'Histoire de la Médecine, this is probably a site for the more serious devotees of medical education and history. Like Montpellier University, this contains a serious collection of original manuscripts and reproductions of many of the most famous treatises in the history of medicine. Visitors must register as library users (this is still the main medical school library) and can then access the very easily navigable computer search engine, even though it is only in French. The medical history section is in a lower floor vault, with its own dedicated librarian who is very knowledgeable. Security is tight and access to the more valuable items is restricted. The collection is mostly in Latin and French, with occasional Greek, but no English-language editions are to be found here.

Examples of documents to be found here include Hippocrates's *Aphorisms*; the *Regimens Sanitaria* from Salerno; the complete Galen; and Pasteur's *Maladies de Vers* and other treatises. If you can read Latin or French, enjoyment is assured. If not, the drawings, diagrams and depictions of diseases are still interesting

Location: School of Medicine, 12 rue de l'École de Médecine, 75006, Paris (6E).

Easiest access: Odeon Metro station (Lines 4 and 10).

General interest to medical history:		★☆☆☆☆	
Relevance to medical education history:		★★★★☆	
Ease of access:		★★★☆☆	
Tourists		*Researchers*	X

6.8. Pasteur Museum, Paris

Louis Pasteur is revered in France as one of the greatest medical researchers of all time. His is an interesting story. He began as a physicist interested in crystallography and used microscopes to examine them, as these were becoming more powerful and more accessible. While Director of Science in Lille (northern France), he made accidental observations of wine fermentation and worked

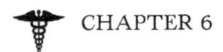
CHAPTER 6

out that lactic fermentation, a process that ruins wine, was an active process from contaminating elements. He was the first to observe many common bacteria, drawing them because there was no photographic equipment at the time.

This is a well-maintained museum that is primarily about Pasteur's scientific discoveries. However, it is worth considering the impact that his discoveries had on the way in which medicine was practised and taught. From his work came the concepts of sterilisation and early vaccine development. Both have had a huge impact on the way in which health care is provided and health professionals are taught. Here lies much of the early development of preventative medicine.

Location: 25 rue du Docteur-Roux, 75015, Paris (15^E).

Easiest access: Pasteur Metro station (Lines 6 or 12) or a 15-minute walk from Gare du Montparnasse.

Website: www.pasteur.fr/fr/institut-pasteur/musee-pasteur

General interest to medical history:		★★★★☆	
Relevance to medical education history:		★★☆☆☆	
Ease of access:		★★★★☆	
Tourists	X	*Researchers*	

6.9. Library of the National Academy of Medicine, Paris

This is the headquarters of the society for medical history in France and houses copies of some of the older manuscripts, including copies of Vesalius' original manuscript in Latin.

Access is difficult, as the library closes for much of the summer period, when tourists are more likely to visit. Further, the society is most interested in visiting scholars or researchers. Intending visitors should seek access well in advance and be prepared to show proof of their academic status, particularly if they want access to the rarer pieces in the collection. An ability to speak French is probably essential.

Probably for only the serious researchers.

Location: 16 rue Bonaparte, 75006, Paris (6^E).

Easiest access: Saint-Germain-des-Prés Metro station (Lines 4 or 10).

Website: bibliotheque.academie-medecine.fr/

General interest to medical history:	★☆☆☆☆	
Relevance to medical education history:	★★★★★	
Ease of access:	★☆☆☆☆	
Tourists	*Researchers*	X

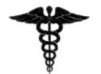

CHAPTER 7:
ENGLAND

It may come as a surprise to many in the English-speaking world that what is now the United Kingdom was not a leader in medical education and practice until much later than the rest of Europe. Until the Middle Ages, England, Scotland, Wales and Ireland were a series of small domains with varying degrees of cooperation and organisation (one might ask how much this has changed!). These were frequently disrupted by invasions by other groups, such as the Romans, Vikings and Normans and it was arguably not until relative stability was achieved that medical practice developed locally. Much of the development was in or around London, the site of wealth and source of international trading influence. After the Norman invasion, most qualified medical practitioners were Paris-trained, although some came from Italian or even Arab influences.

England had two early universities – Oxford and Cambridge. Both were dominated by the Catholic Church, as were most early European universities. Both began with a philosophical approach based on Aristotle's writings. Medicine was traditionally studied as a postgraduate course after studying the arts. There were few teachers, most of whom were also members of the clergy, and there was little of the European tradition of teachers also running thriving private practices for the wealthy. There were also few students, partly because the universities mainly taught theology and the classics, and partly because students had to pay high fees (although they might be sponsored by a wealthy family, friends or benefactors). The two universities were also fiercely competitive from the outset. Oxford predated and influenced the development of the Paris school, because during the early years of the universities, English Kings ruled in parts of France. French and English approaches later diverged substantially.

Many of the interesting developments in medical education took place not at the great universities, but in the private guilds that governed the medical profession, mostly in London, but also in Edinburgh and other large commercial centres. The focus appeared to be less on standards than on protecting income and political influence. Three dominant groups emerged: university-educated physicians, who diagnosed and treated illnesses based on symptoms, the humours and astrology; apprenticeship-trained apothecaries, who practised healing through medicines; and apprenticeship-trained barber surgeons, who bled patients, lanced boils and amputated limbs. Competition within and between these three groups often led to conflict, and sometimes violence. All three groups were supported by the general population, the wealthy and royalty. Many practitioners used techniques from all three groups – possibly the original general practitioners – but by around the eighteenth century the concept of medical specialisation emerged. The move to specialisation was not as rapid as in France and Germany and was even resisted by a profession dominated by generalists – not just general practitioners, but also general physicians and surgeons. Medical specialists did not become common in the United Kingdom until the second half of the twentieth century.

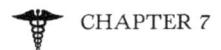 CHAPTER 7

Despite the absence of riches found in Greece, Italy and Montpellier, there are many interesting historical sites to visit and reflect on how medicine developed as a profession. Fortunately, most are very accessible and not far from popular tourist pathways. The sites are listed in approximate historical sequence in each location but may be visited in any order.

The Medical History Society of London has a lot of information on several medical museums in London, including some not discussed here. Their website is: www.medicalmuseums.org.

7.1. Wellcome Galleries, Science Museum, London

The best place to start in the UK is with a very interesting modern museum that provides a succinct summary of the development of international medical practice, from ancient times to the present. Many visitors to London will go to the Science Museum anyway, as it is a great museum that covers many fascinating technological developments that make up the modern world. Here can be found Stephenson's Rocket, and some of the wonderful machines that powered the industrial revolution in Victorian Britain. The Wellcome galleries are on the first floor of the main building and include information relevant to medical education amidst a series of displays about the development of medical technology. Perhaps surprisingly, the galleries include one of the few collections of objects used in Mesopotamian and Egyptian medicine; British archaeologists were obviously very active in the land we now know as Iraq, where pre-Hippocratic medicine has its roots. Curated content varies from time to time.

Beyond the Wellcome Galleries, the museum houses collections relevant to medical science in several other places. The emphasis is on technological development, but here and there can be found displays of medical items, mostly of more recent times. There are also displays of Greco-Roman, Islamic, Chinese, Indian, Arabic and traditional North American medicine, providing a brief overview of the international development of medicine. Displays change regularly, but there is always something to see in this museum.

Location: Exhibition Rd, Kensington, London.

Easiest access: South Kensington Tube station (Circle, District and Piccadilly lines)

Website: www.sciencemuseum.org.uk

General interest to medical history:		★★★★★
Relevance to medical education history:		★★★☆☆
Ease of access:		★★★★☆
Tourists	X	Researchers

7.2. Oxford University

It is hard to leave Oxford University out of a guide to sites relevant to the history of medical practice and education, but much of Oxford's medical fame emanates from the recent past, with a focus on the history of scientific discovery, which (although interesting) is not the focus of this book. Oxford is a university that is a small city and contains a wonderful array of interesting buildings and museums. It is not difficult to spend a day or two just taking in the obvious sites. However, tracking down sites that illuminate the early development of medical education and practice requires a bit of work.

Oxford was the first university in England, claiming to have commenced teaching in some form in 1096 and growing with royal support over the next century when Henry II banned English

CHAPTER 7

scholars from attending the University of Paris. A Royal decree formally established the university in 1248. It was based on the European universities of the time, and so was primarily concerned with teaching theology, law and the arts. Unlike most universities, Oxford is a federation of colleges, within which most of the real educational development and power lies. Medicine was introduced in some early colleges from about 1240 and taught by theologian medical practitioners trained mainly in Montpellier and Italy. There were very few formally trained medical practitioners at the time and most provided services to the wealthy and powerful. Early medical education initiatives were regarded as being more vocationally oriented, meaning that students (usually members of religious orders) were taught the practical skills of medicine more than the underlying philosophy and logic that was coming out of the southern European schools. The first official Oxford medical graduate was reported in 1312.

The Oxford curriculum required students to acquire an MA (Master of Arts) degree first and then study medicine; the curriculum was a total of eight years, reduced to six where students had previous relevant learning. Theology dominated, as did grammar, rhetoric and logic, all to be taken before embarking on "real" medical subjects such as anatomy and astrology. The number of students was small – only forty in the fourteenth century and fifty-four in the fifteenth century. These low numbers were in part due to a restriction placed by some colleges, either banning the study of medicine (only theology was allowed) or limiting it to one or two Fellows at a time.[1]

The best way to connect with early medical education here is probably to wander around the old town and visit some of the older colleges, absorbing the academic atmosphere. Perhaps start with a climb to the top of Carfax Tower, as this provides a reasonable panoramic view of the centre, where most of the old colleges are located. It was these colleges, rather than the university, that drove academic developments, and young doctors were trained in small groups within the colleges by college staff members, who for several centuries were resident (and celibate) theologians, philosophers and physicians. Access to individual colleges is difficult beyond the parts accessible to the general public, unless a Fellow of the college is known and asked to arrange access to the more private areas such as the libraries, where records of early college activities are likely to be found.

There is also a small collection of old medical and surgical instruments in the basement of the Old Ashmolean Building in Broad Street, which houses the History of Science Museum. Because of the orientation towards scientific discovery, much of the display concerns technical advances rather than medical education. A highlight when I visited was a small special display of old anatomy books from the sixteenth and seventeenth centuries. These include: *Margarita Philosophica*, by Gregor Reisch (1508); *Opera Chirurgica*, by Ambroise Paré (1594); *Catoptrum Microcosmicum*, by Johann Remmelin (1619); *De Humanis Corporis*, by Adrian Spiegel (1632); and *Cerebri Anatome*, by Thomas Willis (1664). The latter has the original drawings of the "circle of Willis".

References

1. Rawcliffe, Carole. *Medicine and Society in Later Medieval England*. Sutton Publishing Ltd, London, 1995.

Location: About 90 km west of London.

Easiest access: Walk from Oxford railway station.

General website: www.oxford.ac.uk.

History of Science Museum: www.mhs.ox.ac.uk.

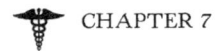

CHAPTER 7

General interest to medical history:		★★★☆☆	
Relevance to medical education history:		★★☆☆☆	
Ease of access:		★☆☆☆☆	
Tourists	X	Researchers	

7.3. Cambridge University

As with Oxford, Cambridge University is a powerful university that has contributed greatly to scientific discovery in medicine and continues to do so. It is well worth a visit to see how one of the great universities functions amidst ancient buildings and the resources won through its success. Like Oxford, Cambridge is a federation of powerful independent colleges and much of the history lies with the early colleges. The architectural and artistic features make the trip to Cambridge worthwhile. However, as with Oxford, there is also little to see easily that is immediately relevant to the early development of the medical profession in England. One of the most interesting aspects of the *Oxbridge* connection is the rivalry between Oxford and Cambridge. This rivalry is as old as Cambridge University, established in about 1209 and granted a royal charter in 1231 by Henry III as England's second university. Medical studies were first recorded in about 1270.

As at Oxford the course was long, based on theology and the classics, and restricted to relatively small numbers of students – only fifty-nine medical graduates are recorded during the fourteenth and fifteenth centuries.[1] There seems to be long gap in the documentation from the Middle Ages, even though the university became eminent in medical scientific discovery, particularly during the eighteenth and nineteenth centuries.

This may be because, although Cambridge University formally established its medical school in 1842, the clinical school at Addenbrookes Hospital became a major teaching site relatively late, when a complete medical school program was established in 1976. For the period between the old college-based education and this recent development, the university provided a traditional, science-based pre-medical course, after which graduates would enter clinical schools, often in London, often in class groups that blended Cambridge and London students. This may explain the virtual absence of apparent interest in medical practice in the Cambridge sites.

As with Oxford, the best way to explore the history of medical education in Cambridge is to visit the whole town, particularly if you have friends with connections. Each of the older colleges has a rich history in which medical training played a small part. The town is compact and easily walked, so the older colleges are easy to visit, at least at a superficial level.

There are also some obvious sites to include in any visit. The first is the Whipple Museum, which includes a wide range of displays relevant to the development of science. A small part of this is relevant to medical science, but very little to medical education. The other site is the main university library, which possesses a collection of original medical journals since their inception in the nineteenth century, as well as some older manuscripts. Unfortunately, accessing the library collection is difficult for people without a Cambridge connection and prior arrangement.

References

1. Rawcliffe, Carole. *Medicine and Society in Later Medieval England*. Sutton Publishing Ltd, London, 1995.

Location: 120 km north-east of London.

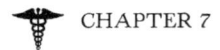

CHAPTER 7

Easiest access: Walk (20 minutes) or bus from Cambridge railway station.

Website: www.cambridge.ac.uk

General interest to medical history:	★★★☆☆
Relevance to medical education history:	★★☆☆☆
Ease of access:	★☆☆☆☆
Tourists	X	Researchers	

7.4. St Bartholomew's Hospital Museum, London

Readers of medieval mysteries will often find mention of a house of healing in the eastern end of the city of London. This is most likely to be the original St Bartholomew's, arguably London's oldest hospital, established in 1123 by Rahere, who was nursed back from the brink of death by monks in Rome. On his return to London, he established a priory and hospital dedicated to St Bartholomew, who appeared in a vision and chose Smithfield, a marshy area near several poor London suburbs and an often-used site of public execution. At the time there were few doctors, and little could be done to help most victims of disease and injury that were brought in for the care of their souls. Under Rahere's guidance, St Bartholomew's attracted monks with skills in the use of herbs and other medicinal plants, and developed a reputation as a house of healing, rather than just a house of death.

While there is a small historical museum on site, just walking around the hospital is an interesting experience, as many older buildings have been preserved or added to. The museum includes displays about the history of the hospital and the development of medieval practice. Sadly, some were destroyed in World War

II bombing. There is a copy of the original royal charter from Henry I, dated 1133, and plans of the early buildings, when the hospital mainly offered rest with clean air, food and water. However, hospital staff learned much from observing the volume of work that the hospital attracted and wrote several treatises on contemporary medical practice, including Mirfield's *Breviarium Bartholomei* (1395), a compendium of diagnoses and remedies for a wide range of commonly experienced fevers and chills. All three groups of health professionals – apothecaries, physicians and surgeons – worked here in apparent harmony.

The hospital's reputation grew and attracted many famous physicians and surgeons to its mostly voluntary medical staff, many of whom helped the needy here as a charitable duty while charging their wealthy patients high fees. One example is William Harvey, who worked out how blood circulates and published *De Motu Cordis* in 1628. Another was Percivall Pott, whose classic description of an ankle fracture was based on his own! Some claim that the discipline of pathology began here, based on the observations of hospital staff, and this was one of the first places to perform general anaesthesia in the 1840s. This hospital grew into one of London's largest and most famous teaching hospitals, although it has been re-structured as central London's medical schools amalgamated and hospital services were rationalised.

Location: West Smithfield Place, London.

Easiest access: Barbican or Farringdon Tube stations

Website: www.bartshealth.nhs.uk/st-bartholomews-museum-and-archives

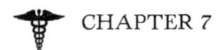
CHAPTER 7

General interest to medical history:		★★★★☆
Relevance to medical education history:		★★★☆☆
Ease of access:		★★★★☆
Tourists	X	*Researchers*

7.5. The Old Operating Theatre and Herb Garret, Guy's Hospital, London

Just south of the River Thames and very close to the city is the site of the original St Thomas's Hospital, one of the oldest in London. First mentioned in documents dated 1212, the hospital was closed in the 1870s and moved to Lambeth when London Bridge was rebuilt. Part of the original hospital was re-discovered in 1956 in the attic of the hospital church. The church had been part of the original priory that became the hospital but reverted to the cathedral after the move. The building housed the original nineteenth century surgical theatre, first used for teaching in 1821, and an herbarium and medicine-making facility that was in use 300 years ago. Both have been faithfully restored to their original design.

Entry to the museum is via a narrow, winding fifty-two-step staircase into the garret (tower) – do not bring large or heavy bags with you for this visit! The old operating theatre has a central flat area containing an operating table, surrounded by five U-shaped tiers on which apprentices and students could stand and observe. Public patients would normally have their operations performed in lesser facilities by apprentices but would allow students to watch if this brought a senior surgeon to the case, as this probably increased their chance of survival. The roof has a large skylight so that the surgeons could see what they were doing, at least on sunny days. For darker days there was a gas-powered overhead theatre light.

The associated display of old surgical instruments is testimony to the rather gruesome nature of surgery in the nineteenth century, when anaesthesia was both ineffective and dangerous and death rates were high from either pain or infection. The wealthy would avoid having surgery in places like this, but rather bring the surgeon to their homes, where surgery on the kitchen table was associated with fewer infections and a higher chance of survival, although no less pain. Aseptic techniques and better analgesia did not come until the mid-nineteenth century. This theatre was the site of the first use of general anaesthesia in 1846.

The juxtaposition of the herbarium and operating theatre is intriguing, as until relatively recently physicians, apothecaries and surgeons had different origins and training and did not often cooperate. The former would use astrology, bloodletting and herbs to cure disease, while the latter would use sharp instruments rapidly and without analgesia. The herbarium display is a little more interactive than the operating theatre, as it is possible for visitors to mix a medicinal paste from herbs and oil and produce pills of approximately equal size (if not dosage), using original equipment from the time. The links to aromatherapy are easy to see here as many of the herbs and plants used have a pleasant smell that might boost the spirits of the patient, or at least mask the foul odours of the dying. The bookshop has some wonderful historical books for sale.

Location: 9a St Thomas St, London.

Easiest access: London Bridge Tube station (Northern and Thameslink Lines).

Website: oldoperatingtheatre.com/

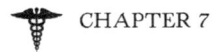

CHAPTER 7

General interest to medical history:	★★★★☆	
Relevance to medical education history:	★★★☆☆	
Ease of access:	★★★★☆	
Tourists	X	Researchers

7.6. The Worshipful Society of Apothecaries, London

Ever wondered where the United Kingdom's traditions of using herbs and other plants as health agents came from and how they were related to medical practice? As a major trading centre even before the Roman invasion, London was the source of exotic herbs and spices from other parts of the world and so traders along the River Thames became pivotal in the supply of herbs thought to have medicinal properties.

In the thirteenth century the Grocers Guild was formed to manage the production of, and trade in, herbs and other natural medicinal agents, but most members were traders rather than health professionals. Gradually a new group emerged from within the grocers, the Guild of Pepperers, who specialised in the use of exotic herbs and spices mixed in special concoctions as medical treatments. First recorded in 1180, this group came to regard themselves as a distinct group of health professionals, capable of diagnosing ailments, manufacturing medicines and dispensing these medicines either directly to the public, for a consultation fee, or on the advice of physicians. They remained a powerful trading group, controlling the importation and trade of essential ingredients, as well as selling confectionery and perfumes. They were popular with royalty, who appointed personal apothecaries to keep them well, and with commoners, because they were more accessible and much cheaper than physicians. At the time physicians often used astrology and other mystical arts and did not mix medicines, and surgeons belonged to a separate Company. There was often conflict between the three groups, particularly between physicians and apothecaries, with several prosecutions of apothecaries for acting as "unregistered" physicians.

Aiming to achieve recognition equal to that of physicians, the apothecaries in 1607 became a separate section of the Grocers Company. In 1617 they broke their ties with the fruit and vegetable dealers to form their own professional organisation, the Worshipful Society of Apothecaries, with a charter signed by King James I. Premises were obtained in a former Dominican Priory close to Bridewell Palace and the trading docks on the River Thames. From here they maintained their control on the trade in spices and cultivated relationships with royalty. The original building was destroyed in the Great Fire of London in 1666 and then rebuilt as the current Hall, which was added to during the nineteenth century. The building alone is worth a visit, with its great halls, art collection and an archive that includes records back to 1617 and a library of current medical books. At their peak the apothecaries had their own medicines factory adjacent to the Hall and, just along the river, a small farm growing unusual medicinal plants – the Chelsea Physic Garden. The garden no longer has this purpose but is open to visitors. It is an easy walk from Sloane Square Tube station.

This organisation evolved into one of the most important health professional groups in the United Kingdom, winning their battle with the physicians, with the help of royal patronage and the refusal of physicians to stay in London and tend those struck down by the plague. They were responsible for the standards of medicines dispensed in London and provided increasingly formalised training in the medicinal arts, with heavy emphasis on botany and what later became pharmacology.

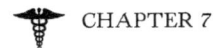

In 1815 they were granted the right to hold licensing examinations for medical practitioners. In some ways Society members were the forerunners of today's general practitioners, rather than pharmacists. The licensing examinations later bestowed a formal qualification – the Licence in Medicine and Surgery of the Society of Apothecaries or LMSSA – which was recognised until 2008 as equal to a university medical degree. The Society has also pioneered the development of some specialties through establishing a range of postgraduate Diplomas. Some of these resulted in new specialties. For example, the Diploma in Midwifery evolved into membership of the Royal College of Obstetricians and another Diploma led to the development of Occupational Medicine as a specialty. More recently the Society has introduced formal Diplomas in military medicine, Medical Jurisprudence (for Police Surgeons or Government Medical Officers), medical history and genitourinary medicine. Hence this 800-year-old group has had a profound influence on medical education in the United Kingdom.

The building also contains an interesting library that included documents dating back to their early days. This is mainly for researchers, but I found the staff to be very helpful.

Further reading

Hunting, P. *A History of the Society of Apothecaries.* The Society of Apothecaries, London, 1998.

Location: Black Friars Lane, London.

Easiest access: Blackfriars Tube station (Circle, District and Thameslink Lines)

Website: www.apothecaries.org; www.chelseaphysicgarden.co.uk/

General interest to medical history:		★★☆☆☆
Relevance to medical education history:		★★★★★
Ease of access:		★★★★☆
Tourists	X	*Researchers*	

7.7. Hunterian Museum, The Royal College of Surgeons of England, London

Perhaps the most interesting micro-history in London is that of the development of the profession of surgery. It began as the lowest status group, perhaps because of the high death rates prior to general anaesthesia. The group in society that was practised with using knives were the barbers. In addition to cutting hair and shaving beards (a few were also rumoured to be contract assassins!), some would also, for a fee, lance a boil, cut a vein to bleed patients and attempt to cut out abnormal, infected or gangrenous flesh. It is uncertain how much the ancient surgical arts, such as trephination, were practised by barber surgeons in England. Some patients went directly to barber surgeons, others were referred by physicians or apothecaries.

Friction developed within the barbers and the more medically oriented established a separate guild to differentiate them from mere barbers, and the first Master of the Company of Barbers was sworn in during 1308. In response to the friction between surgeons and physicians, a historic attempt was made in 1423 to amalgamate the two groups in the new College of Physicians and Surgeons, but this lasted only a year. The barber surgeons formed a separate Guild of Surgeons, with membership limited to about twenty. In 1435 the identity was formalised, and a coat of arms was adopted. In 1493, surgeons and barbers signed an agreement to formally separate and acknowledge their different roles: surgeons would not cut hair and barbers would not perform operations, except for pulling teeth.

Henry VIII formally granted a charter to the Company of Barber Surgeons in 1540, largely because he wanted a secure supply of surgeons to assist in his military campaigns, where surgeons were the most useful members of the medical profession. Injuries were terrible and often the only way to deal with them was by amputation and excision of damaged flesh. An interesting part of the deal with Henry VIII was that the surgeons were guaranteed the annual supply of the corpses of four felons, executed at the nearby Newgate prison. This was to foster the study of human anatomy, partly in response to Vesalius' pioneering work at Padova and to ensure that educational standards were maintained.

The uneasy relationship between barbers and surgeons continued until 1745, when Surgeons formed their own Company and members agreed to practise only surgery. This caused some problems as many members had been "general practitioner–surgeons", supplying apothecary, physician and surgeon services. In 1800 the Company became the Royal College of Surgeons. Throughout this period the main method of training was through apprenticeship, with no formal curriculum or assessment required to become a member of the college. There was conflict with both the apothecaries and the physicians over who should license general practitioners, as all three had examinations and licensing certificates; one route was Membership of the Royal College of Surgeons (MRCS). Training in anatomy was particularly difficult, with bodies having to be obtained from the "resurrection men" who, for a fee, exhumed bodies from graves. Recognising that the annual supply of four legal bodies was insufficient, an Act of Parliament in 1832 made legal the supply of bodies to medical training institutions, by now established in newer medical schools. In 1843 the College established a more formal training pathway with an examination that was in two parts – basic sciences and clinical sciences – both employing written papers and oral examinations.

The building in Lincoln's Inn Fields was planned during the late eighteenth century in response to the donation of the Hunter collection. This was completed in 1813, but was too small and rebuilt in the 1830s. It is an impressive building, with a grand front of columns. Inside there are two areas for visitors – the Hunterian Museum and the library. The library is in a magnificent two-level hall and contains a large collection of historical books and manuscripts back to the early nineteenth century.

As with all the libraries mentioned in this book, the visitor needs to know what to look for. I was interested in documents about education and the role of artists and was not disappointed. I was able to see an original 1625 article of indentureship to a surgeon, a 1777 apothecary's bill (very expensive for the era!) and wonderful collection of original artworks by A.K. Maxwell, vividly depicting injuries from World War I. At this time artists were the most reliable recorders of visual images, and here can be seen drawings and paintings of terrible head and neck wounds, with the results after surgery, and of mustard gas injuries. A particularly poignant feature is the inclusion of the patient names, battalion and sometimes whether or not they survived. The librarians were very helpful.

Further reading

Blandy, J.P. and Lumley, J.S.P. *The Royal College of Surgeons of England: 200 Years of History at the Millennium.* Royal College of Surgeons of England, London, 2000.

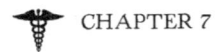
CHAPTER 7

Cohen, Bertram. "King Henry VIII and the Barber Surgeons. The story of the Holbein cartoon." *Annals of the Royal College of Surgeons of England*, 1967, vol. 40, pp. 179–94. Reprinted with revisions by RCSE.

Location: 35–43 Lincoln's Inn Fields, London.

Easiest access: Holborn station (Central and Piccadilly Lines).

Website: www.rcseng.ac.uk/museums-and-archives/hunterian-museum/

General interest to medical history:		★★★★☆	
Relevance to medical education history:		★★★★☆	
Ease of access:		★★★★☆	
Tourists	X	Researchers	

7.8. Royal College of Physicians of England, London

The physicians were arguably the most traditional and successful group of medical practitioners during medieval and Renaissance England, but they faced stiff competition. Physicians were trained at Oxford and Cambridge in relatively small numbers and so were the only group with a university education. They studied the humanities and philosophy, as well as the works of Galen and Hippocrates. They focused on understanding diseases, diagnosing them and giving advice on management, which often relied on herbal remedies. Some also studied anatomy, generally by travelling to Padova or Montpellier, and a few dabbled in surgery and even dispensed herbal medicines. Most had relatively few clients who were usually wealthy, as their services were expensive. They also considered themselves to be above the barber surgeons and apothecaries, who were not university-trained and whose organisations were commercial trading guilds. However, patients generally made choices on whom to see first and most could not afford a physician.

As with the barber surgeons, Henry VIII formalised the organisation of physicians by granting a charter to the Royal College of Physicians of London in 1514. It seems that he wanted both kinds of practitioners, as well as apothecaries, to coexist, as each had a different role. Henry VIII was very keen to gain the help of the physicians during the plagues that were rife at the time. The original College building was in Knightrider Street, very close to the Apothecaries' Hall.

The physicians had a pre-eminent role in medical education, as they were the best connected to the educational establishment. They were the first group to establish funded academic positions in Oxford and Cambridge and therefore assumed a dominant position in medical schools. The College could also licence medical practitioners through what developed into a Licentiate examination (the Licentiate of the Royal College of Physicians or LRCP). This was independent of the other licensing processes for many years, although more recently was delivered in collaboration with the apothecaries until recognition by the General Medical Council ceased in 2008.

The current College building dates from the 1980s and the architecture is suitably contemporary. In keeping with the College's education profile, the building is an active and successful educational centre, with a large lecture theatre and several seminar rooms that appear to be in almost constant use. The most striking feature is the artwork as there are several portraits of College luminaries throughout the building. There is also a small library on the second floor, but this does not particularly welcome

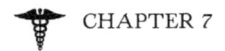

CHAPTER 7

casual visitors. Its collection is mostly about current medicine and College affairs; very little dates from earlier than the eighteenth century. When I visited the staff were not particularly interested in discussing the history of medical education with a non-RCP visitor. Researchers should make prior contact.

Further reading

Clark, G. *A History of the Royal College of Physicians of London.* Clarendon Press, Oxford, 1964.

Location: 11 St Andrews Place, Regents Park, London.

Easiest access: Regents Park, Great Portland and Warren Street Tube stations (Bakerloo, Circle and Victoria Lines).

Website: www.rcplondon.ac.uk/

General interest to medical history:	★★☆☆☆
Relevance to medical education history:	★★☆☆☆
Ease of access:	★★☆☆☆
Tourists	*Researchers* X

7.9. Florence Nightingale Museum, London

One of the most enduring images of nursing is that of Florence Nightingale holding a lamp as she tended soldiers in the Crimean War. As important as this was, it is arguably the least important aspect of the work of this truly remarkable woman, because she had a major impact on three issues relevant to health care and healthcare education.

The first is that she made it acceptable for well-educated young ladies to become nurses. At the time nursing was a low status job, more related to cleaning and pandering to the whims of surgeons, probably making little real contribution to patient care. One early description used the words "ignorant, illiterate, drunken and immoral". Recruits came from the lower classes of society and their training was rudimentary. Florence was a rather refined young lady, a well-educated member of a wealthy family. She travelled widely as a young adult and developed a religious conviction to do good for society. Overriding her parents' wishes she chose nursing, studying in a German hospital. On her return to London she was recognised as a leader and became superintendent of a small hospital, an honorary position made possible by family support. The next year, 1854, saw her volunteering to lead a group of trained nurses to tend to the injured in the Crimean War.

The second is that she was a gifted pioneer of public health research, as she observed, collected data on and then published influential reports about the appalling condition of English hospitals, particularly military hospitals, which were dark, disease-ridden halls of misery and suffering. Injured patients would lie in agony with no attention to dressings, infection control or pain relief. She produced reports that included statistics and pie charts to support her conclusions. These data were so impressive and powerful that they resulted in changes in the role of nurses, professional relationships between surgeons and nurses and the design of hospitals. She developed the concept of open, airy hospital wards with a window for each bed, a design that can still be found in older hospitals in the British-influenced world. One of the first hospitals influenced by her principles was the new St Thomas's Hospital adjacent to the museum. The decision to move it away from the noisy re-developed London Bridge was also her idea, based on an analysis of where most patients lived and the potential noise levels. Sadly, many recent hospital designs have not maintained her principles!

CHAPTER 7

Her third impact was in nurse education, as she designed a form of nurse training that included educational standards, a formal health science curriculum, apprenticeship training and examinations. Nurses now managed patients and wards, with doctors visiting to provide medical advice. This model has only recently changed in the developed world, with nursing moving to the university sector, and indeed continues in many parts of the world. Her first "Nightingale School" was established in 1860 at the newly re-constructed St Thomas's Hospital, adjacent to the museum.

The easy-to-find museum has displays that span her life and major contributions, including the original books and reports she wrote. There is a twenty-minute video that provides an interesting overview.

Location: 2 Lambeth Palace Rd, just south of the Westminster Bridge.

Easiest access: Waterloo Tube station (Northern, Jubilee and Bakerloo Lines)

Website: www.florence-nightingale.co.uk

General interest to medical history:		★★★☆☆	
Relevance to medical education history:		★★☆☆☆	
Ease of access:		★★★★☆	
Tourists	X	*Researchers*	

7.10. Great Ormond Street Hospital for Children, London

The interest in this hospital relates to its role in the development of emerging specialties in child health for doctors and nurses. The hospital was established in a cottage by Dr Charles West, who worked almost exclusively with women and children. The population of London had grown quickly during the industrial revolution and the health system just could not cope with caring for the poor, particularly children. Children occupied very few hospital beds in general hospitals but accounted for a large proportion of deaths, particularly from epidemics of infectious diseases.

Assisted by a committee of benefactors, the hospital opened in 1852 in a cottage in Great Ormond Street with just ten cots. It was so popular and so busy that it grew rapidly, not so much because children could not be cared for in other hospitals, but because the Great Ormond Street Hospital developed a particular child-centric approach. This developed into a way of caring for children that lead to the development of nurse and medical education programs that became essential for nurses and doctors who wanted to work in paediatrics anywhere in the United Kingdom. Funding has always been an issue here, as it was developed as a free service to the poor and had to survive on charity. The hospital managed to find some strong support over the years. Charles Dickens and Oscar Wilde held readings of their books in well-subscribed festival dinners, which became very popular with London's wealthy set. Another famous author, J.M. Barrie, donated the royalties of his book and play, *Peter Pan* in 1929, and this was continued in perpetuity after the usual 50-year period by a special Act of Parliament. This copyright continues to be a source of income.

There used to be a small museum across the road known as the Peter Pan museum. It was rather difficult to access and now the collection is dispersed throughout the hospital. There is a

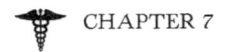
CHAPTER 7

Peter Pan Gallery with paintings and statues and memorials to the paediatricians who pioneered the development of a range of specialty paediatric services, including orthopaedics, ear nose and throat, ophthalmology and oncology.

The message from Great Ormond Street is that only a specialist children's hospital can really care for sick children. The hospital still uses the argument to support its battle to remain an independent hospital. Other children's hospitals opened but few survived the mergers of the late twentieth century. Regardless of how strongly you accept this notion, caring for children is a special part of health care and the hospital is a special place.

Location: Great Ormond Street, St Pancras, London.

Easiest access: Holborn Square Tube station

Website: www.gosh.nhs.uk

General interest to medical history:		★★★☆☆	
Relevance to medical education history:		★★☆☆☆	
Ease of access:		★★★☆☆	
Tourists	X	Researchers	

7.11. Anaesthesia Heritage Centre, London

Although the development of safe general anaesthesia allowed the development of modern surgery and made possible the kind of safe surgical procedures that we now take for granted, the role of anaesthetists was poorly recognised for several decades. They were just one of the surgeon's assistants, not as well paid and certainly not receiving much attention.

Early images of surgeons at work show conscious, terrified patients being held down while a surgeon amputates limbs with what appear to be carpenter's tools. The more quickly the surgeon removed the limb, the better. Survival rates were low due to pain and blood loss, and there was not much available for post-operative analgesia. Attempts to develop analgesia relied on drugs, typically opium and alcohol, and even compression of limb nerves to produce a temporary loss of sensation. The world's first demonstration of safe inhalation anaesthesia was provided in October 1846 by W.T.G. Morton in Massachusetts General Hospital, followed in December that year in England. The uptake was rapid, and soon there were many providers of anaesthesia, but they struggled for recognition and remuneration and felt poorly treated by the surgeons. In 1893 they formed a Society for the Study of Anaesthesia and this became the Association of Anaesthetists of Great Britain and Ireland, the group that hosts this museum.

This small, but modern, museum provides an interesting, short tour through the development the early equipment and of the science and technology that makes anaesthesia so safe today. There is also a small library that includes early descriptions of the development to the technology and the profession of anaesthesia, but it contains very little about the period prior to the formation of the Association and the interesting professional tensions of the time.

Further reading

Boulton, T. *The Association of Anaesthetists of Great Britain and Ireland 1932-1992 and the Development of the Specialty of Anaesthesia: Sixty Years of Progress and Achievement in the Context of Scientific, Political and Social Change.* Association of Anaesthetists of Great Britain and Ireland, London, 1999.

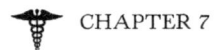

CHAPTER 7

Duncum, B. *The Development of Inhalation Anaesthesia.* Oxford University Press, London, 1947. Reprinted Royal Society of Medicine Press, London, 1994.

Location: 21 Portland Place, London.

Easiest access: Oxford Circus, Regents Park and Great Portland St Tube station Open: During normal office hours, but an appointment is recommended.

Website: anaesthetists.org/Home/Heritage-centre

General interest to medical history:		★★★☆☆	
Relevance to medical education history:		★☆☆☆☆	
Ease of access:		★★★☆☆	
Tourists	X	*Researchers*	

7.12. London (Royal Free Hospital) School of Medicine for Women

Rather than visiting a building, consider having a quiet lunch or snack in the park in Tavistock Square, central London, to reflect on a remarkable advance in medical education. In the south-eastern corner is a statue to the memory of Louisa Aldrich-Blake (1865–1925), a well-known surgeon and pioneer of the role of women in medicine. At a time when almost all medical practitioners were men, and few women could gain entry to a medical school, she was not only an early graduate, but also the first female to gain postgraduate qualifications in surgery. She became a leading hospital surgeon and later, Dean of the London School of Medicine for Women. The park is just 200 metres from where the original medical school buildings were located in Handel and Hunter Sreets.

The tale is fascinating now, when women medical students often outnumber men and the role of women in medicine is well established, even if not all challenges have been overcome. The monastic university model of medical education excluded women from studying medicine for several centuries, although there are reports that the school at Salerno admitted women as students and teachers.[1] Until the late nineteenth century, British women who wanted to study medicine had to go abroad, usually to the USA. Once licensed there, they could return and practice medicine in their home country. A few managed to gain entry to Edinburgh in the early 1870s but were expelled on the basis of their gender. These determined individuals managed in 1874 to set up their own medical school in London – the London School of Medicine for Women (LSMW), with friendly male doctors providing tuition and the Royal Free Hospital providing the clinical experience.[2] The School's developers were influenced by the developments on the other side of the Atlantic, in Boston, where several medical schools for women flourished after the first – the Boston Female Medical College – opened in 1846. Indeed, by 1860, eighteen per cent of Boston's medical practitioners were women.[3]

Aldrich-Blake entered the new London School in 1887 and graduated in 1893 with the Gold Medal for surgery. The barriers to female medical professional life remained substantial, as postgraduate training posts and hospital positions were usually reserved for men. Despite this, Aldrich-Blake obtained a Master of Surgery in 1894 and entered surgical practice. She had a distinguished career as a surgeon at the Royal Free Hospital, with the military in France during World War I, and served as Dean of the LSMW from 1914 until her death in 1925, the year she was made a Dame of the British Empire.

The LSMW grew and prospered as demand for places increased. However, the surrounding world changed slowly, and it was not until 1947 that all medical schools in the United Kingdom became

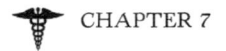

co-educational. That was when the LSMW admitted male students and became the Royal Free Hospital School of Medicine. Since then several amalgamations have seen it become part of a large central London medical school, the Royal Free and University College Medical School.

While many would argue that women's rights still have a way to go to achieve equality with men, the early medical women were pioneers who achieved a great deal, well before they were allowed to vote. Hence, they were at the forefront of profound societal change, and the Aldrich-Blake memorial is a fitting reminder of this era.

References

1. Puschmann, T. and Hare, E.H. *A History of Medical Education*. [Translated and edited by E.H. Hare] Facsimile of 1891 ed. Hafner, New York 1966.

2. Bell, E. Moberly. *Storming the Citadel: the Rise of the Woman Doctor*. Constable, London, 1953.

3. Walsh, Mary Roth. *"Doctors Wanted: No Women Need Apply". Sexual Barriers in the Medical Profession, 1835–1975.* Yale University Press, New Haven, 1977.

Location: Tavistock Square, London.

Easiest access: Russell Square Tube station (Piccadilly Line)

General interest to medical history:		★★☆☆☆
Relevance to medical education history:		★★★★☆
Ease of access:		★★★★★
Tourists	X	*Researchers*

7.13. Alexander Fleming Laboratory, London

This museum has a special connection with Australians because, while Alexander Fleming accidentally discovered the origin of the antibiotic penicillin, the final stage of development was completed by the Australian, Howard Florey. Fleming's most important contribution to medical science was actually the discovery of lysozyme, a natural chemical found in human secretions that can inhibit bacterial growth, but the accidental discovery of penicillium mould is what he is somewhat reluctantly remembered for. He left a Petri dish on a bench while he went away on a holiday, and on his return noticed that a culture of staphylococci was inhibited by penicillium spores. However, he did not realise the significance of this discovery, believing that penicillium spores may be toxic to human life, and sat on the information for thirteen years.

The addition to his research team of Howard Florey – the Australian connection in this tale – resulted in the information coming to light. Florey was working on the antibacterial use of lysozyme in infections resistant to the recently discovered sulphonamides. He re-discovered notes on Fleming's earlier accidental findings on penicillium spores and worked with Ernst Chain (a German fleeing the Nazis) to establish the active ingredient in brewer's yeast broths. Word War II provided the backdrop and the driving force for this research, as surgical treatment alone was not ideal for wounds with established infections and there were high rates of amputations and deaths. The identification of the pure active ingredient – penicillin – changed the way infections were managed and improved patient outcomes both during and after the war.

Hence this story is not so much one of a magnificent research project that ran true, but one of accidental discovery, based on

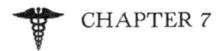

CHAPTER 7

careful observation, of a substance that was to have a profound effect on medical practice and on medical education. Up until this discovery treating infections was difficult and based on hygiene measures and surgery; afterwards medical practice began to use antimicrobial agents in ever-increasing amounts and varieties, and non-surgical medical practice became more prominent.

At this historic site visitors can climb up a rather narrow staircase to a reconstruction of Fleming's original laboratory, complete with old microscopes, Petri dishes, the original documentation and his awards for contribution to science. The materials are focused on the earlier work with lysozyme, rather than the more famous penicillin outcome, but the atmosphere is interesting as it conveys a sense of what it must have been like to work in laboratory research in the 1920s and 1930s.

Location: Corner of Praed Street and Norfolk Place, Paddington, London, UK.

Easiest access: Paddington Tube station (District, Circle, Bakerloo, Metropolitan and Hammersmith & City Lines).

Website: www.imperial.nhs.uk/about-us/who-we-are/fleming-museum

General interest to medical history:		★★★☆☆
Relevance to medical education history:		★★☆☆☆
Ease of access:		★★★☆☆
Tourists	X	Researchers

7.14. Bethlem Museum of the Mind, London

Medical students used to learn very little about chronic mental health conditions. In some medical schools the breadth and depth were defined by a visit to some form of "institution for the insane". These were terrible places where people with serious, long term problems were detained "for their own protection" and provided with accommodation, food and a form of supervision. Some received specific medical treatment, but most were beyond medical understanding and were just locked away from polite society. Worryingly, many had conditions that are now relatively easily managed in the community, such as epilepsy and thyroid disease. Even more worryingly, physical and sexual abuse was not uncommon as most staff had no health professional training. Psychiatry did not exist, and medical care was based on restraining people, usually physically, sometimes chemically. Most chemicals prescribed were toxic. Most people were scared of the residents, who were generally called "lunaticks". Most were probably harmless to others, but there have been some famous exceptions. The service was closer to a prison than a healthcare facility.

The value of this museum is that it documents carefully, although briefly, about 700 years of mental health care in a relatively wealthy, sophisticated society. The original Bethlem was north of the Thames River, at Moorgate, just within the old city of London and not far from the Tower of London. It was founded and sponsored by a few benevolent wealthy Londoners to care for the poor souls who had lost their minds and tended to roam the streets and become ill through malnutrition and violence. While there was an element of "out of sight, out of mind" about this benevolence, there was at times strong support from the upper classes because mental health (then and now) knows no social class barriers. Many residents were from the wealthier, upper classes; some were gifted writers and artists.

CHAPTER 7

The quality of the medical care was not always high. While some medical practitioners were great leaders and pioneers, others were cruel and incompetent. This variability was because the medical posts were not often regarded as attractive. Hence care was often provided by part-time doctors who mostly focused on private practice. The fortunes of the hospital fluctuated over the centuries, with periods of sound leadership, management and health care, interspersed with periods of the opposite. Some rather famous "criminally insane" people were sent there, and some doctors conducted experiments on inpatients and their bodies. The name was often shortened to "Bedlam", a word that has become synonymous with chaos and disorder. It was moved and rebuilt twice nearby, once in an impressive building designed by Sir Christopher Wren. It was moved in 1815 south of the river to what is now the Imperial War Museum in Southwark, and then in 1930 to a semi-rural location that is now a major London psychiatric hospital.

The museum collection has two parts. The first is the historic documentation of the hospital during its phases of existence. This includes paperwork for individual patients, minutes of meetings and plans for the buildings on the various sites. There is also a small display of physical restraining devices – mostly leather straps – that were the common forms of management. The second, perhaps more interesting, part of the museum is a collection of artworks by some of the hospital's more famous residents – Richard Dadd and Louis Wain, from the late nineteenth and early twentieth centuries, respectively. Both were accomplished artists with strong followings during their life. There are also works by lesser known artists. Some provide interesting insights into the minds of the artists, with clear evidence, beautifully expressed, of mental anguish.

A visit to the museum is best accompanied by a walk along Bishopsgate to Liverpool Street Station, the approximate original thirteenth century site. This provides a sense of the East End location and its proximity to other central London institutions.

Further reading

Arnold, C. *Bedlam: London and its Mad*. Simon and Schuster, London, 2008.

Location: Monks Orchard Rd, London, Beckenham, Kent BR3 3BX

Easiest access: Train from Victoria to East Croydon or Charing Cross or Waterloo to Eden Park Station (Line to Hayes in Kent), then a bus or a short walk.

Website: museumofthemind.org.uk/visit

General interest to medical history:		★★★☆☆	
Relevance to medical education history:		★★☆☆☆	
Ease of access:		★★★☆☆	
Tourists	X	*Researchers*	

7.15. Freud Museum, London

On the wealthier north side of London lies an interesting contrast to the mental health care documented at Bethlem. Regardless of one's views on psychoanalysis, Sigmund Freud was a great pioneering psychiatrist. Fleeing the Nazi regime, he left Austria in 1938 and moved to London. He was eighty-two years old and this was to be the last year of his life. He was in poor health and upset at having to flee, so his children tried to re-create the atmosphere of the original house in Vienna, using the same furniture and organising the rooms in a similar way. The "real" Freud museum is actually in Vienna, where his family home is filled with pictures and writings from his early life through to his flight to London (see Austria 4). Here in North London, while living rather quietly, he continued to see some patients and write about psychoanalysis and his hobbies.

And, yes, here is his original analytic couch, although no, you may not lie on it. The rooms are set up just as when he was there, with a consulting room within his study. Here he would listen as patients voiced their thoughts in "free association", and he would interpret these thoughts. Surrounding the desk, chair and couch is an amazing personal collection of archaeological antiquities, predominantly from Egypt and Greece but also some from China. He was a keen amateur archaeologist and managed to collect some rather valuable pieces. Visitors can also see the library, which houses a substantial collection of books that reflect his interests in art, history and philosophy, as well as his medical books. Throughout the house are works of art either owned by Freud or with some connection to Freudian history or themes. Freud often made connections between psychoanalysis and the insights gained from reading and appreciating culture and art.

One of the more interesting aspects of Freud's life was his contribution to medical education. He pioneered a form of psychiatric case presentation, in which patients would speak about their concerns in front of an audience of therapists and students. This form of clinical discourse was regarded as both therapeutic for the patients and a source of learning for medical students and psychiatrists.

The ambience of the house is reserved and scholarly, in keeping with the man and his influence. One of the highlights is the small bookshop on the ground floor overlooking the delightfully English back garden. Here is an amazing collection of academic discussions about Freud, his colleagues and their theories. Most members of the psychoanalytic movement were Jews, and this explains much of the Nazi hatred of them. In Germany their books were destroyed, and psychoanalysis was derided as a "Jewish science". I was surprised to see several books devoted to criticism of psychoanalysis on the grounds of philosophy, politics and religion, just as there were books extolling its virtues and almost worshipping Freud. The staff were helpful in explaining some of the complex history.

Location: 20 Maresfield Gardens, London.

Easiest access: Finchley Rd Tube station (Jubilee and Metropolitan Lines).

Website: www.freud.org.uk

General interest to medical history:		★★★☆☆	
Relevance to medical education history:		★★☆☆☆	
Ease of access:		★★★☆☆	
Tourists	X	Researchers	X

7.16. Wellcome Trust, London.

This is the headquarters for one of the largest pharmaceutical companies in the world. Among their more altruistic endeavours is one of the most comprehensive medical history libraries in the world. The focus is on original books that have made a difference to medical practice, rather than just a collection of contemporary textbooks, so here you may find very old editions

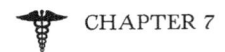

that you will see cited often but are generally unavailable. This is one of the few locations of English translations (as well as Latin and Greek versions) of manuscripts by early greats such as Galen and Hippocrates, as well as manuscripts by pioneering English medical researchers.

Visitors must register in order to gain entry, choosing between either a day pass, ideal for a casual visitor, or three-year membership, more useful for academics or frequent visitors. The collection covers two floors of the building and is clearly categorised and organised; I had no difficulty in navigating the collections. Catalogues can be searched online, and internet access can be booked for extended searches. Visitors may not photocopy any materials; staff members provide a photocopying service with a half-day turnaround, but this is relatively expensive. There is also a small display of an interesting aspect of medical history: when I was there the theme was the concept of death greeting dying patients, based on fascinating old manuscripts.

This library is a must for those with a serious interest in medical history. The online catalogue is excellent, so it is both easy and desirable to search for materials of interest before visiting. It also offers something for almost everybody because the collection is so broad and accessible. The entrance hall houses rotating exhibitions that highlight some aspect of medical history for the general public.

Location: Central London, UK.

Easiest access: Euston Square (Circle) or Warren St (Piccadilly Line) Tube Stations.

Website: wellcomecollection.org/

General interest to medical history:	★★★☆☆
Relevance to medical education history:	★★★★★
Ease of access:	★★★★☆

Tourists	X	*Researchers*	X

7.17. Eyam, Derbyshire

While many interesting sites are located in London, one of the most intriguing in the United Kingdom is about 250 kilometres from London and might not be on many itineraries. Eyam is a small town, perhaps more of a village, about half an hour by road south-west of Sheffield. This is the site of a memorial to the plague of 1665, marking arguably the first recorded recognition of the concept of isolation as a means of limiting the spread of contagion. There are other "plague villages", but this is one of the most notable.

Europe was struck by several plagues over the centuries, some of which killed a substantial proportion of the population. The history of the plagues records different symptoms, transmission methods, infectiousness and mortality, so it is possible that there was more than one cause for the disease referred to as the "Black Death".[1] The most common cause is thought to have been the bacterium *Yersinia pestis*, transmitted by rat flea bites. *Yersinia pestis* was discovered only in the late nineteenth century and is known for certain to have caused only the most recent plagues. Infected people developed fevers, haemorrhagic swellings called "buboes" and most succumbed within days. At the time nobody understood what it was or how it spread, except for a vague notion of "evil air".

CHAPTER 7

One day in this small village George Viccars, the tailor, became ill with what appeared to be the plague. He died four days later with the tell-tale signs. It was postulated later that a flea must have travelled from London in a bolt of cloth, although recent analysts believe that this is unlikely. When the diagnosis was made, panic set in and many wanted to flee the village.

However, the parish priest, the Reverend William Mompesson, called the village folk together and suggested a different strategy. He postulated that the disease was already among them and that fleeing citizens would in fact spread the disease to their friends and family in other villages. He proposed that the village seal itself off from the outside world, letting in and letting out no- one, thereby limiting the spread of the disease.

Perhaps surprisingly, the village folk agreed. In those days, villages were relatively self-contained as communication and travel were limited. The word was spread that the village was being isolated, although it is thought that several villagers escaped, and it is rumoured that the Reverend Mompesson secretly sent his children away. However, most people stayed and faced their futures. Food was bought by leaving money at a site on a hill above the village, where outsiders left provisions in exchange. This all sounds rather similar to strategies used during the COVID-19 epidemic in 2020!

Over the next few weeks, most of the villagers went down with the disease and an appalling seventy-three per cent (257 out of about 350) died, including the Reverend's wife. After about a year the plague appeared to have died out and the village reopened. It is not known if the isolation did limit the spread of the disease, or if it increased the death rate in this village, as the plague was common in the area at the time.

The village is now a memorial to this brave act of voluntary quarantine. The churchyard is worth a visit to see the record of deaths and the rows of graves. The road through the village is worth the walk as each cottage has plates that list who died and when – people in rows of cottages appeared to fall ill in sequence as the disease moved along the road. At the far end of the road is a small museum that provides an interesting and detailed history of the tragic events.

References

1. Cohn, S.K. *The Black Death Transformed: Disease and Culture in early Renaissance Europe.* Hodder Education, London, 2003.

Location: Derbyshire, UK, between Sheffield and Manchester, along the A623.

Easiest access: Preferably by car, but bus tours are available.

Website: www.eyam-museum.org.uk/

General interest to medical history:		★★★☆☆	
Relevance to medical education history:		★★☆☆☆	
Ease of access:		★★☆☆☆	
Tourists	X	*Researchers*	

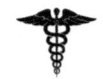

CHAPTER 8:
SCOTLAND

Scotland is considered separately from England because of its history and the roles that Scotland has played, in its own right, as a centre of medical education. There are five medical schools in Scotland and there are more medical student places per head of population than the rest of the United Kingdom. The Scottish schools provide examples of both ancient and venerable (St Andrews), innovative (Dundee) and research powerhouse (Edinburgh). Scotland educated women doctors much earlier than did England. An unusual feature of the five schools is the way that they work closely with each other, and with the National Health Service in Scotland, in developing and delivering medical education.

Edinburgh is a fascinating old city with a proud tradition of providing medical education. By the eighteenth century, Edinburgh was regarded as a centre of development in medical practice. The old town of Edinburgh has three sites where this relatively recent history can be explored, but in chronological order the tour should start at St Andrews.

8.1. University of St Andrews

St Andrews was established in 1413 as a university town, much like Oxford and Cambridge, and lays claim to having the third oldest university in the English-speaking world. The university is the heart of the community even today, as the surrounding town has not developed as much as Oxford and Cambridge have. The current medical school was established in 1897 but medical students may have trained there since 1450. The model of medical education is also unusual, rather like Oxford and Cambridge were until about fifty years ago, in that the course is a three-year pre-medical only course, from which students graduate with a first degree. They then move to other Scottish schools or Manchester University for clinical education, after which students are awarded a second degree. St Andrews and Dundee Universities recently established a collaborative, graduate entry, more community-based course.

Visiting the town is really the same as visiting the University and the medical school. All students live in the town and can walk to all facilities, which are close to both the harbour and an old castle. The town exists to serve the needs of students and staff of the university, as well as the adjacent world-class golf courses. There are several old buildings that are worth a visit, if they are open, but otherwise a visit here is really an opportunity to experience the student town atmosphere.

Location: St Andrews, Fife.

Easiest access: By car, parking difficult. Also train to Leuchars, (8 km), then taxi.

Website: www.st-andrews.ac.uk

General interest to medical history:		★☆☆☆☆
Relevance to medical education history:		★★★☆☆
Ease of access:		★★☆☆☆
Tourists	X	*Researchers*

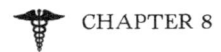
CHAPTER 8

8.2. Museum of Scotland, Edinburgh

The Museum of Scotland houses some exhibits of general interest to medical history, in addition to a large collection of things related more broadly to Scotland, but finding them is not necessarily easy. On the third floor is a small collection relevant to medical practice, mostly focusing on the development of "male midwives" whose work evolved into the discipline of obstetrics. The most interesting exhibit is probably a sedan chair used by a successful obstetrician. A sedan chair, carried by at least two men, was a way of keeping some separation from the rest of humanity, partly for privacy and partly to appear successful. Midwifery was originally not a high-status job, but its practitioners aspired to higher things.

Location: Chambers Street.

Easiest access: An easy walk from the city centre.

Website: www.nms.ac.uk

General interest to medical history:		★★☆☆☆	
Relevance to medical education history:		★★★☆☆	
Ease of access:		★★★★☆	
Tourists	X	*Researchers*	

8.3. Royal College of Surgeons of Edinburgh, Edinburgh

Around the corner in Nicholson St is Surgeons Hall, which houses two collections in the headquarters of the Royal College of Surgeons of Edinburgh, founded in 1505. Unlike in London, apothecaries and surgeons in Edinburgh were allies. In the 1770s, the modern medical school was established, with both surgeons and physicians collaborating.

The public exhibition demonstrates the development of surgery from the Middle Ages to the present. Local surgeons feature prominently, as does a strong connection with military campaigns, which generated many surgical innovations. Until the late eighteenth century surgeons and physicians were competitors, with their own training schools. Access to Playfair Hall requires booking, due to the sensitive nature of some of the material on display. This is worth it to see the series of prints by Sir Charles Bell, who during the wars of the Napoleonic period painted carefully detailed, yet somehow more holistic, representations of soldiers with wounds to limbs, head or the abdomen, with annotated descriptions of the cases. One of the most powerful is of a man dying of tetanus, in an arched-back spasm that matches the textbook descriptions. These paintings were used as teaching aides, another example of the synergy between art and medical education.

Location: Nicholson Street.

Easiest access: An easy walk from the city centre.

Website: www.rcsed.ac.uk/the-college/surgeons-hall-museums

General interest to medical history:		★★★★☆	
Relevance to medical education history:		★★★★☆	
Ease of access:		★★★☆☆	
Tourists	X	*Researchers*	X

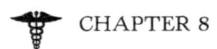

8.4. Anatomical Museum, University of Edinburgh

Around another corner, in Teviot Place, is the Anatomy Department Museum, a working teaching facility for the medical school and open on select days only. Among the microscopes and modern models to be found in most medical schools is the skeleton of the infamous Burke, who was sentenced to "hanging and dissection" for illegally providing cadavers for anatomy teaching. This is a fascinating connection to the nearby nether region of the city called Cowgate, a seedier area famous in novels for dubious businesses and crime.

Alexander Monro was the first Professor of Anatomy who pioneered the teaching of anatomy by demonstration dissections. His sessions were so popular that not even the brisk rate of nearby criminal executions could avoid a shortage of cadavers, so some enterprising morticians took to grave robbing. Monro opposed this trade, but it continued – even keen medical students were rumoured to resort to this to improve their learning. Munro's observations provided clear descriptions of disease processes that led to advances in surgical treatment. The small hospital for the indigent and ill that he began in 1729 grew to become the Royal Infirmary, now a major teaching hospital designed by the famed Edinburgh architect William Adam. Anatomy maintained its dubious reputation for about 100 years, when the above-mentioned Burke and his accomplice Hare were convicted for murdering people to sell their bodies to Edinburgh anatomist Robert Knox.

Location: Teviot Place.

Easiest access: An easy walk from the city centre.

Websites: www.ed.ac.uk/visit/museums-galleries/anatomical

General interest to medical history:		★★☆☆☆	
Relevance to medical education history:		★★★★☆	
Ease of access:		★☆☆☆☆	
Tourists	X	Researchers	

CHAPTER 9:
CZECH REPUBLIC

The current Czech Republic is another part of Europe that has been at the junction of cultures and languages, this time German and Slavonic, has suffered domination by several different empires, and has often been at the centre of political action. During the early Middle Ages, most of the country was within the Holy Roman Empire of the German nation. Prague was one of the more dominant German-speaking centres, with a strong tradition of literature, the arts, architecture and cultural life. It was also the location of the first medical school in Germanic Europe, in a university founded in 1347 by Papal Bull issued by Pope Clement VI with three faculties – liberal arts, theology and medicine. As with other German universities, the founding was a response to problems in the Roman Church, where the French had become independent and appointed their own Pope. The university was named Charles University, after the Bohemian King and Holy Roman Emperor Charles IV, although the name has varied over the centuries. The first intake of medical students was probably in 1348, into what is now called the First Faculty of Medicine.

Because of the mix of languages and cultures, Charles University was unusual in that, depending on the strength of Jesuit control, it often ran courses in several languages. In the Middle Ages, the language of teaching medicine at Charles University was Latin; later, during the Austrian Monarchy, it was German; since 1833 the students have been taught in Czech. In 1992 teaching of medicine in English was commenced as a program in parallel with the Czech-taught courses and aimed at both local and international students wanting to work in English-speaking countries.

The main value of a visit to Prague is the broader history of an often-conquered country that maintained its own strong sense of identity and culture. There is relatively little available that is specifically related to medical education, but the broader cultural exhibits do offer brief glimpses on medical practice and student life in Prague. One example of this is the rich literary history. Franz Kafka is remembered in a museum bearing his name, and he wrote a series of short stories under the title *A Country Doctor*. The city has a tradition of a sometimes unusual artistic culture (the origin of the word "Bohemian") and has been central to middle European political development. Students in Prague have often been at the forefront of cultural and political developments. There is a small collection of medical equipment from the Czech Medical Association located in a small house at the back of the National Library, but access to non-Czech speaking visitors is difficult.

9.1. First Faculty of Medicine, Charles University, Prague

The medical school still exists as one of three medical schools managed by the Charles University. Strangely, very little is open for visitors. I could not find a medical history museum, at least nothing in English. Some old medical school buildings remain, but these are mostly from the last 200 years, with nothing remaining from its earlier history. Most of the buildings are not identified as historical sites, perhaps because they are surrounded by the much

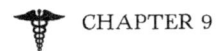

more historic and attractive buildings that are everywhere in this beautiful city. All visitors can do is walk the streets of the old city, absorb the atmosphere and imagine what life as a medical student in a middle European city.

Location: Ovocný trh 5, Praha 1, 116 36, Czech Republic.

Easiest access: Any transport to the old city centre and just walk the streets

General interest to medical history:		★★☆☆☆	
Relevance to medical education history:		★☆☆☆☆	
Ease of access:		★★★★☆	
Tourists	X	*Researchers*	

9.2. National Museum, Prague

One of the few medical-related museums in Prague is a small but elaborate museum of pharmacy, maintained as part of the National Museum, which is really a network of small, specialist museums. As elsewhere in central Europe, the role of the apothecary and the development of homeopathy was strong in Prague, and this museum is a reconstruction of an apothecary, both manufacturing and retail. There is a range of measuring and cooking equipment, herbs and other ingredients, bottles and flasks. The shop front is an attractive display of timber shelves and storage jars from which the apothecary could make up a mixture.

Location: Nerudova 23, Mala Strana, Prague

Easiest access: Palace access road, near the top Nerudova Street. The nearest Tram stop is Malostranske Namesti and the nearest station is Malostranska.

General interest to medical history:		★★☆☆☆	
Relevance to medical education history:		★★☆☆☆	
Ease of access:		★★★★☆	
Tourists	X	Researchers	

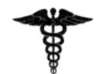

CHAPTER 10:
AUSTRIA

Vienna is another of those European cities that should be on any travel itinerary, with its well-preserved architecture and a vast range of music and art museums. However, this is not just a centre for classical musical culture, but also the location of one the earliest modern medical schools in Europe, the second in German-speaking Europe after Prague. The university was founded in 1365 by Duke Rudolph IV, under the patronage of Pope Urban V. Its structure was similar to that of other early European universities, teaching mostly theology, philosophy and law in separate faculties. Medical education began in the early fifteenth century, with anatomy dissection demonstrations by staff from Padova and the establishment of the House of Physicians. However, medical education remained theoretical until a clinical medical school was formally established in 1754 at the nearby general hospital.

This was a very conservative university, remaining dominated by Jesuit thinking until the late eighteenth century, when Protestants were admitted and instruction in German was allowed. When the new medical school was opened, human dissection was not going to be allowed, so the university acquired a collection of wax models from Florence. However, as Jesuit control waned, human dissection was allowed in an anatomy dissection theatre that was built in 1784.

The University of Vienna medical school flourished as an independent centre of medical research and education. As with German medical schools, the emphasis has been on serious scientific research, rather than innovations in medical education. Medical students and practitioners will almost certainly know at least two famous names from here. The first is Semmelweis, who died of septicaemia from a hand wound suffered while an inpatient of a mental asylum. Rumour has it that he allowed the wound to become infected in order to prove his controversial observation that patients died less often of puerperal fever when under the care of midwives who washed their hands, compared with doctors who did not. The second is Billroth, who pioneered several modern surgical procedures.

All of the places of interest in Vienna are either within or close to the original university and general hospital, so visiting them is easy in a city with such good public transport and the scenery to make the walk interesting. Three of them are in the Josephinum building, part of the original medical school, but now a collection of museums and the academic Department of Medical History, as well as a few other academic groups. The main university campus is itself worth a visit, as it has several garden courtyards between faculty buildings, making it a very attractive inner-city campus.

10.1. Museum of Medical History, University of Vienna

This is a good place to start, as the collection is so accessible and of such general interest. The main focus is on the history of the local medical school and its more outstanding personalities. There is an interesting display of early surgical equipment, notes and photographs of local scientific discoveries, and the nucleus of a larger and less accessible dermatology display. The focus of the collection is relatively recent, as the clinical school began in 1785.

The main attraction is the large range of wax models that were made in Florence in order to replace human dissection as a teaching and learning tool. This is the largest such collection on display in the world. It includes several life-sized models of the entire skeletal, muscular and vascular systems. The most famous is known as the "Venus", a woman reposing on a couch wearing a pearl necklace, opened up from neck to pubic area, and with removable thoracic and abdominal organs. In addition, there are almost 200 hundred, smaller (yet usually life-size) models of all organs, joints and more-or-less everything that anatomists might want to display. They are in full colour, so are much more authentic than formalinised dissection materials.

It is interesting that these models were hardly ever used for teaching, because by the time they arrived, regulations had been relaxed to allow human dissection. However, they are of such quality that they would still be very useful learning tools.

Location: First floor, Währingerstraße 25, Vienna.

Easiest access: An easy walk from the inner-city centre, just west of the Schottenring, part of the ring road around the old centre. The nearest U-Bahn station is Schottentor-Universität (U2, 600 m).

Website: www.josephinum.ac.at/en/

General interest to medical history:		★★★☆☆	
Relevance to medical education history:		★★☆☆☆	
Ease of access:		★★★★☆	
Tourists	X	*Researchers*	

10.2. Picture Archives, University of Vienna

The Department of Medical History houses a collection of photographs, sketches and paintings relevant to medical history. Most of the collection concerns the history of the local medical school, but there are also images relevant to other medical schools in Europe. As with most academic collections, one needs to know what one is looking for, although the curator is extremely helpful and welcoming to visitors with a genuine interest. If a visit is planned, make contact before arriving in Vienna and indicate your interest. The most interesting collection is the original coloured drawings that go with each of the wax models in the history museum. These are remarkably clear and realistic drawings that label the relevant anatomical features, so these were a major part of the teaching collection. They cannot be displayed openly because of their fragility.

Entry is by appointment only, so check the university webpage for details.

Location: Second Floor, Währingerstraße 25, Vienna.

Easiest access: An easy walk from the inner-city centre, just west of the Schottenring, part of the ring road around the old centre. The nearest U-Bahn station is Schottentor-Universität (U2, 600 m).

Website: www.josephinum.ac.at/en/

General interest to medical history:	★☆☆☆☆
Relevance to medical education history:	★★★★★
Ease of access:	★☆☆☆☆
Tourists	*Researchers* X

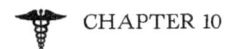 CHAPTER 10

10.3. Library and Manuscript Collection, University of Vienna

This is another one for the serious visitor, and access has to be arranged in advance. If you are seriously interested in old manuscripts and copies of classical manuscripts, you should take this step. The collection of old manuscripts is in a small but wonderful room with shelves up to the twenty-foot ceiling, but the catalogue is simple to follow. I was able to see four 500-year-old versions of Vesalius' classical anatomy book, the *Canons* of Avicenna, aphorisms of Maimonides and the *Regimens Sanitas Salernitum*. Most of the older manuscripts are in Latin, some are in French (from Montpellier), the more recent are in German and occasionally English. These are treasures that do not often see daylight and must be handled with gloves.

The library is on the ground floor, and it offers a more traditional collection of books and journals relevant to the history of medicine. It has a very good index of authors, titles and subjects. As with all of the libraries in the old European medical schools, it helps to speak the local language, and here knowledge of German makes searching much easier. Again, the staff were very helpful.

Entry is by appointment only, so check the university webpage for details.

Location: Ground Floor, Währingerstraße 25, Vienna.

Easiest access: An easy walk from the inner-city centre, just west of the Schottenring, part of the ring road around the old centre. The nearest U-Bahn station is Schottentor-Universität (U2, 600 m).

Website: www.josephinum.ac.at/en/

General interest to medical history:	★★★★☆	
Relevance to medical education history:	★★★★★	
Ease of access:	★☆☆☆☆	
Tourists	Researchers	X

10.4. Sigmund Freud Museum, Vienna

This museum is a memorial to the man and his interests in psychoanalysis. Unlike its smaller counterpart in London (see England 15), this has enormous detail of his life from childhood in a small country town to his flight to freedom from Nazi persecution. Almost all signage is in German, although an audio guide is available in several languages. Perhaps due to the language barrier, I saw less that was relevant to the history of medical education than in the London museum, but this museum still offers interesting insights to one of recent medical history's more famous and controversial leaders. There is little of the original furniture (that appears to be in London), but hundreds of photographs and documents on the walls of what was Freud's consulting room and study. The museum shop also sells copies of his major works in several languages, as well as books about the controversy that continues to surround psychoanalysis in Austria.

Location: First Floor, Berggasse 19, Vienna.

Easiest access: By foot, about 300 metres off Währingstraße, close to the Josephinum. An easy walk from the inner-city centre, just west of the Schottenring, part of the ring road around the old centre. The nearest U-Bahn station is Schottentor-Universität (U2, 600 m).

Website: www.freud-museum.at/en/

General interest to medical history:		★★☆☆☆
Relevance to medical education history:		★☆☆☆☆
Ease of access:		★★★★☆
Tourists	X	*Researchers*

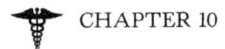

10.5. Federal Pathological-Anatomical Museum, Vienna

The most interesting aspect of this museum is the building. It is an unusual round building of four levels, located in the rear corner of the grounds of the main university teaching hospital, almost hidden by some tall trees. The reason for its position and design is probably the original role for the building – the first psychiatric hospital for the city, known as the "madhouse". Constructed in 1784, it resembles a prison more than a hospital, as each floor is a ring of small rooms off a circular corridor. The role changed after almost 100 years to become an accommodation building for hospital staff, so they could be close to work. One can imagine the parties they must have held there!

Since 1971, the building has housed the Federal Pathologic-Anatomical Museum, a very large collection of specimens from the hospital's pathology department. As with similar collections elsewhere, the collection reflects the changing patterns of disease and the development of medical knowledge over the last 200 years or so, as illustrated through the specimens that were collected and maintained. The focus is on the scientific advances in Germany and Austria in the microbiology of infectious diseases (mainly tuberculosis and sexually transmitted diseases) and orthopaedics (early prosthetic developments), with images, gross specimens and wax models. There is also an interesting section on the teaching of phrenology and craniometry, a practice developed by Franz Joseph Gall in Germany that was popular in the early nineteenth century.

Location: Narrenturm, at the rear of the University campus, Spitalgasse 2.

Easiest access: By foot, through the University campus off Alser Straße. A comfortable walk from the inner-city centre. The nearest U-Bahn station is Schottentor-Universität (U2, 800 m).

Website: www.nhm-wien.ac.at/narrenturm

AUSTRIA

General interest to medical history:	★★☆☆☆
Relevance to medical education history:	★☆☆☆☆
Ease of access:	★★★★☆
Tourists	X	Researchers	

CHAPTER 11:
GERMANY

Germany has a proud and dominant place in the history of medicine, but not so much medical education. There are records of early medicine, as practised by wandering Goths and Vikings.[1] The first medical schools in German-speaking Europe were in Prague and Vienna. Soon after, a split in the Catholic Church saw German medical students evicted from the Paris school, and so in 1386 the Roman Pope Urban VI established the first medical school in what is now Germany, in Heidelberg. For the first hundred years or so the teaching was entirely theoretical, with no clinical teaching until about the late fifteenth century, when a clinician was appointed to augment the philosophical teachings of Hippocrates, Galen and Avicenna. Early records indicate that enrolments were small for four or five centuries. Advances in medical education in Germany were later than elsewhere in Europe. For example, human dissection was not used until the middle of the seventeenth century. The great age of German medicine arose in the eighteenth to twentieth centuries, when Germany arguably dominated the development of the scientific and technical basis of medicine. As a result, most of the medical history museums in Germany focus on science, not education.

Perhaps because of the widespread destruction during World War II, there is not much from the past left to see in modern Germany. Most of what is left to display is really about scientific research, at which Germany has excelled. For example, just one Berlin university has produced twenty-nine Nobel Prize winners, and German names are commonly found attached to discoveries and developments in pathology, microbiology, neurology and orthopaedics.

The history of medical education in Germany is closely linked to this tradition of scientific discovery, as a strong foundation in science was arguably best developed in Germany. The more vocational or practical aspects of medical education were not strong, and indeed are still not. Class sizes are large and the tuition mostly theoretical. Until recently many German medical students still relied on international elective placements to gain clinical experience; this has now changed, and a stronger practicum is now mandatory. Medical degrees are not awarded until after a small research thesis is submitted and marked. Further, passing a medical licensing examination is required to achieve eligibility for registration as a medical practitioner.

The chosen sites begin with the beautiful city of Heidelberg, the location of the third medical school in German-speaking Europe after Prague and Vienna. Thankfully, Heidelberg was largely untouched by World War II, although the castle shows serious damage from a war in 1689! Probably all visitors to Germany should come here to see the wonderful old city, with its narrow, pedestrianised, cobbled streets and the famous castle up on the hill. There are many museums and art galleries in which to pass a couple of days.

The location then changes to Berlin, the ancient capital that recently resumed its status as the capital of re-unified Germany. The Berlin sites are almost all in the section known as Berlin Mitte, the old city centre that was East Berlin until 1989. All are within reasonable walking distance of many hotels and can be reached via an excellent coordinated transport system of underground and above-ground railways, as well as trams and buses. Sadly, perhaps because of its location in one of the developed world's most fought-over cities, there are not many places to visit that are intact or even re-constructed, that are relevant to medicine and medical education. The city is well worth a visit to see its strengths: German culture; the futility of war; the horror of the Holocaust. One aspect of the development of the medical profession that is quite evident here is the inappropriate, and tragic, complicity of some medical practitioners in the Holocaust. Perhaps all should see this and reflect on a role that the medical profession should never again adopt, but I will focus on the more positive developments. Finally, an interesting museum in northern Germany is listed.

References

1. Puschmann T. and Hare, E.H. *A History of Medical Education.* [Translated and edited by E.H. Hare] Facsimile of 1891 ed. Hafner, New York 1966.

11.1. University Museum, Heidelberg University

The University Museum is not particularly focused on the Faculty of Medicine but does record nicely the early history of the university, which was modelled on the University of Paris and had three founding faculties – theology, law and medicine. The university was established following a split in the Catholic Church, which for a while had two popes. Germany's leaders supported the Roman Pope, rather than the French Pope, and so German students and teachers had to leave Paris. The university was established by the Roman Pope, Urban VI, to train faithful Germans. It opened in 1386 and the Faculty of Medicine was first mentioned in documents in 1388; other German Catholic universities had opened already in Vienna and Prague. The faculty remained small for around a hundred years, with just one teacher until a second was appointed in 1482. Students could join at age fourteen and then spend up to eight years to achieve a medical degree. Teaching was mostly theoretical up until the mid-sixteenth century, when the importance of some clinical teaching was recognised. Hence Heidelberg was the first German medical school to offer integrated theoretical and practical learning. Human dissections on executed felons began in 1655. The 1700s were tough times, with wars and closures, but in the early 1800s medical education took a step forward with the opening of a large teaching hospital close by. The 1850s saw the beginning of a very successful period of scientific discovery, with several instantly recognisable names including Bunsen (as in burner) and Henley (as in loop of) followed by four Nobel Prizes for medicine during the last century.

The museum also documents in remarkable detail the rise of national socialism and its impact on higher education in Germany. Some academics supported national socialism, others did not and were sacked; a list of the sacked staff is on display. The main university building was renamed and badged with national socialist emblems, and a senior Nazi was awarded an honorary PhD (a copy is on display).

Much is made of the scientific and technical advances made by the Faculty of Medicine, and of its move in 1974 over the river and downstream to a huge facility in Neuenheimer Feld. There is a scientific medical and zoological museum on the new campus, but the old university is much more interesting.

Two other places in the old city are worth visiting. The first, just around the corner in Augustinergasse, is evidence of the university's early approach to managing misbehaviour. It is open at the same times as the museum, but there is a separate entry and a small additional entry fee), unless you buy the triple ticket to the University Museum. Students who misbehaved (usually drunkenness) were locked up in a special student jail (the Studentenkarzer) for up to four weeks, or until they paid a fine. Inmates spent their time writing poetry on the walls; this can still be read and has even been published in a small booklet. In the current climate of teaching and assessing professionalism in medical schools, perhaps this idea deserves re-consideration? Mind you, there appear to have been several notorious repeat offenders, so it is unclear how successful the approach was.

The second is the former Dominican Friary in Brunnengasse, which was the location of the Anatomical Institute from early 1800s to 1974, when the Faculty of Medicine moved to their new location. It must have taken a sense of either humour or evil to convert a church to a morgue and dissection demonstration rooms! The complex was rebuilt in 1846 in its present form, and it is now used by the Psychology Department. During term times the buildings are open, although the most interesting part – the auditorium in the rounded rear protuberance – is likely to be in use for lectures.

Location: Old University, Grabengasse in the old city area of Heidelberg.

Easiest access: By foot from the beginning of the old city area. Heidelberg itself is about 1 hour by train or bus from Frankfurt. Buses 12, 41 and 42 from the railway station and the more modern city area go right through the Universitätsplatz.

Website: www.uni-heidelberg.de/en/institutions/museums-and-collections/university-museum

General interest to medical history:	★★☆☆☆
Relevance to medical education history:	★☆☆☆☆
Ease of access:	★★★★☆

Tourists	X	Researchers	

11.2. German Pharmacy Museum, Heidelberg Castle

This museum is quite a surprise package, because it is not well advertised, and yet deals well with the European part of the struggle between apothecaries and university-trained medical practitioners (see also Chapter 7, England). The apothecary profession began in the Arab world, probably before Hippocrates, with the first known apothecary claimed to be in Baghdad. The term apothecary seems to be derived from their practice of storing herbs, spices and other plant materials, which would be ground and mixed in many varied combinations to form "natural" remedies. These combinations, or medicines, would be prescribed initially by the apothecary, but later also by physicians, to treat disease. Until medieval times it was widely believed that all diseases were due to an imbalance in the four humours (cold, warm, moist and dry), and the medicines would counteract the humour that was judged to be over-active. Mainstream physicians also adopted similar treatments, and Hippocrates, Avicenna and Maimonides all wrote books listing medicinal treatments based on natural plant ingredients.

The art of the apothecary moved with the spice trade, from the Middle East to Europe and England with traders in the first few centuries of the Common Era. When the Roman Empire collapsed, the secrets of the apothecaries received shelter in monasteries. The art came to prominence again in Salerno, as its multicultural approach to health care flourished (see Italy 3). The first formal definition of the arts of the modern apothecary was the Edict of Melfi, published and promulgated in Italy in 1231.

Just as academic medicine moved from Salerno to Montpellier and into Europe, so too did the profession of the apothecary. It found a strong base in central Germany, where it was taken to new heights, based on German knowledge and skills in chemistry. Minerals and salts were added to recipes, and a wide range of prescriptions were formulated to treat many diseases and maladies. The first German pharmacopoeia was published in 1546 in Nuremberg, not far from Heidelberg. Apothecaries became the dominant German health profession, with large chains of apothecaries setting up branches in most towns, each promoting their own versions of medicines. In competition with the medical profession, apothecaries attended university as early as the eighteenth century, conducted much of the medical research, and even founded what were to become large multinational pharmaceutical companies (Schering, now part of Bayer, is an example). Apothecaries were probably much more respected than general practitioners, who were a rather weak group in Europe. Their influence waned as medicine became the more prominent profession during the twentieth century, probably aided by the persecution of Jews, who comprised a substantial proportion of the leaders of the profession, in the 1930s.

This museum includes an interesting time-sequence display of history, with everything described in both German and English. There are also several displays of what storerooms and preparation rooms looked like in the eighteenth and nineteenth centuries. Some rooms smell quite sweetly of the herbs they contain.

Location: The Otto Henry Building, within the Heidelberg Castle. Entry is through the castle main entrance.

Easiest access: By foot, up a very steep path, or by riding on a cute funicular train, both from just behind the Kornmarkt square. Heidelberg itself is about 1 hour by train or bus from Frankfurt. Buses 11 and 33 go from the railway station and the more modern city area to the Kornmarkt.

Website: www.Deutsches-Apotheken-Museum.de

General interest to medical history:		★★☆☆☆	
Relevance to medical education history:		★★☆☆☆	
Ease of access:		★★★☆☆	
Tourists	X	Researchers	

11.3. Institute for Microbiology and Hygiene, Humboldt University, Berlin

One of the most revered medical scientists in Germany was Robert Koch (1843–1910), a not particularly bright country boy who studied science, then medicine, and developed a passion for delving into dark and dirty places and looking down microscopes in his spare time. He came to national attention when he identified the organism responsible for anthrax, and he was brought to Berlin and given a well-equipped laboratory to help him pursue his exploration of tuberculosis. He was the first to identify the mycobacterium responsible and he announced his discovery at a public lecture in this building on 24 March 1882, a day still recognised internationally. He later devoted his energy to tackling the causes of cholera in the Middle East and malaria in tropical Africa. In 1905 he was awarded the Nobel Prize for Physiology or Medicine. His status in German science is similar to that of Pasteur in France, and the two often competed for attention and funding in their remarkably parallel careers.

The old Institute for Microbiology and Hygiene was housed in an attractive (in a Prussian way) building that managed to survive the bombardment of World War II. The displays are rather inaccessible, as due to funding restrictions there is nobody specifically caring for them. I had to phone several times and had a lot of trouble connecting. This is in fact not really a formal museum, but rather a workspace that has historical value. There are three places here that are worth visiting. The first is the small museum to Robert Koch. Here can be found a collection of photographs and memorabilia from his life, as well as a portrait, a bust, laboratory equipment and the original Nobel Prize certificate. For those with a particular passion for Robert Koch, a visit to the Robert Koch Institute may also be worthwhile, as it contains further information and artefacts, as well as his mausoleum, a setup similar to that for Pasteur in Paris. That is where he did most of his work; he was only ever a visitor to the Institute building.

The second display is the adjacent library room, where Koch delivered his public lecture to an enthralled audience of about seventy people. The room is so small they must have been packed in like sardines. The furniture and decor are the original, and certainly conveys a musty academic ambience. Koch was reputed not to be a confident speaker or teacher, except of research students.

It is the third area, one not even mentioned in the leaflets, that is the most interesting from a medical education perspective, as it reflects a dramatic change in the development of German medical education, and one that has been widely adopted elsewhere. The whole building was designed and built in the 1870s as a new, integrated sciences faculty. Here medical scientists from all disciplines were housed together, primarily for research, but also for teaching, with the rationale that they could learn from each other. In this building a new lecture theatre was built as a "theatre of science", for presentations to students, peers and the general public. The room is steeply tiered so that all can clearly see the speaker and any displays, and there are special terraces for dignitaries round the upper level. Outside the lecture theatre are displays of pathology specimens and wax models of infectious disease rashes. This is a truly remarkable building, as it took the modern scientific era to the people! Sadly, the rest of the integrated facility in adjacent buildings was destroyed by aerial bombardment.

Location: Dorotheenstraße 96, 10117 Berlin.

Easiest access: A short walk from Friedrichstraße U-Bahn and S-Bahn station.

Website: imh.charite.de/en/institute/

General interest to medical history:		★★☆☆☆	
Relevance to medical education history:		★★☆☆☆	
Ease of access:		★☆☆☆☆	
Tourists	X	Researchers	

11.4. Berlin Museum of Medical History of the Charité

This is a modern, well-designed facility that is located within the grounds of the Charité, the large Humboldt University Faculty of Medicine complex that sprawls across several city blocks adjacent to the main city hospital. The complex is an interesting mixture of old and new buildings, named after Rudolf Virchow, the revered "father" of modern pathology and a local medical scientist. His statue can be found near the entrance, on Charité Straße and buildings are named after him.

The museum itself is at the rear of the Pathology building, about 600 metres into the complex. Its collections integrate my three interests: art, literature and medical history. There are three levels above the ground floor entrance. The second level is a space for rotating art exhibitions with a health theme. The third level contains a system-based display of pathology specimens. This is a relatively recent display, with few specimens more than fifty years old, but the material is displayed in an interactive, interesting and informative format that is rarely seen in pathology museums. There are still some rather gruesome exhibits, but they are placed in an appropriate context. The fourth level is a contemporary display of normal pathology, using a combination of models, drawings and interactive computer formats.

The collection is open to the public, with age restrictions (sixteen years and older) to the third level. It is one of the most accessible museums I have seen, as non-professional visitors are likely to learn a lot here. One small problem is that currently everything is in German. This makes reading the displays difficult to study in detail, but most of the material is visual, so visitors without German language should not be deterred.

Location: Schumanstraße 20-21, Berlin 12

Easiest access: A short walk from Friedrichstraße U-Bahn and S-Bahn station.

Website: www.bmm-charite.de/en/index.html

General interest to medical history:		★★★★☆	
Relevance to medical education history:		★★☆☆☆	
Ease of access:		★★★★★	
Tourists	X	*Researchers*	X

11.5. Medical School Library, Berlin

For those with a more academic interest, there are two further places worth a visit. The first is the small medical library that serves the mostly research-focused centres in this complex. Because it is downstairs from the Centre for the History of Medicine, it has a large collection of medical history books. The librarian is helpful and some of the books are in English, but competence in German is required to get the best from a visit. This is a working space for academics rather than a recognised museum, so contact is better made through academic connections.

While in the building, serious researchers should visit the Centre for the History of Medicine, up on the second floor. Although small, this is one of the few centres for academic medical education in the world, and it has been there since 1930. They currently have no information in English, but I found the staff to be very helpful. Prior contact is recommended if visitors have specific questions.

Location: Ziegelstraße 5-9, Berlin.

Easiest access: A short walk from Friedrichstraße U-Bahn and S-Bahn station.

General interest to medical history:		★★☆☆☆
Relevance to medical education history:		★★★★☆
Ease of access:		★☆☆☆☆
Tourists	X	*Researchers*

11.6. Hospital Museum, Bremen

Many visitors to Germany would not think of visiting this smaller regional centre in the north, but Bremen, perhaps surprisingly, is interesting. As part of the old Hanseatic League, it was once a wealthy trading nation-state with strong links to the outside world. There is a rich cultural heritage that is worth exploring, long predating its more recent reputation for industrial development and beer making. Hidden in the grounds of a suburban hospital there is also a small but interesting museum dedicated to the care of the mentally ill from the eighteenth century up until World War II. In keeping with Germany's focus on technological and biomedical development, its efforts to medicalise mental health problems and develop interventions that made patients more easily managed were notable. Highlights include a nasty looking restraining chair, an early electro-convulsive therapy machine and a straitjacket. There is an extensive collection of photographs that depict life in the hospital over the last century or so.

The location is typical of mental health institutions the world over – a rather picturesque setting in a semi-rural area (now an outer suburb). The buildings are attractive, perhaps even relaxing, and it is easy to imagine spending time here recovering from illness in peace and quiet, perhaps even seclusion. This of course reflects the relative paucity of real management options available until relatively recently.

All information is in German only, so visitors without any German proficiency should consider taking a friend who can translate. Most of the exhibits are easily interpreted just by looking, but some of the more subtle exhibits will be missed without the explanations. An example is the material about psychiatry leading up to and during World War II.

An added bonus for visitors is the ground floor art exhibition centre, which runs a series of exhibitions with local artworks, often with some kind of connection to mental health perspectives. There is also a small theatre in an adjacent building for music recitals and plays. The effect of this combination of facilities is that mental health history is presented with strong artistic and cultural links.

The location means that travel times are relatively long (45 minutes from the city centre), but the journey is simple once the correct tram or bus is selected.

Location: In the grounds of Central Hospital East, Züricher Straße 40, Bremen.

Easiest access: From the Hauptbahnhof by S-Bahn Line 1 to Graubündener Straße or bus 24 to Zentralkrankenhaus Ost stop, then a short walk.

Website: www.kulturambulanz.de/kulturambulanz/krankenhausmuseum.php

General interest to medical history:		★★★☆☆	
Relevance to medical education history:		★★☆☆☆	
Ease of access:		★☆☆☆☆	
Tourists	X	*Researchers*	

CHAPTER 12:
HUNGARY

Hungary has a fascinating, often violent history. The dominant culture and language are of the Magyars, who settled in seven waves (the "seven tribes") from near the Ural Mountains area around 896 CE. Visitors may notice that the numbers seven and ninety-six are deeply meaningful in Hungarian culture; they often appear in official labels and names of organisations, buildings and monuments. The history of Hungary is of course much longer than that of the Magyars, as the region has forever been located between Europe and the east, and so has had to survive invasions by the Roman Empire, Attila the Hun, Genghis Khan, the French, the Ottoman Empire, the Austro-Hungarian Empire of the Hapsburgs, Nazi Germany and Stalinist Russia.

Because of the many cultural influences, the current culture is an interesting blend. For example, the culture of the steam baths is very strong, probably because of the Ottoman influence. The cuisine is also different from that of Hungary's eastern neighbours. The language is the most distinctive feature, as Hungarian is from an ancient language that is closest to Finnish and nothing like the main European languages. Gypsy culture is strong and seems to dominate restaurant entertainment. Politically speaking, Hungary has always been a haven for radical thinkers and reformers: most recently in 1956 the city rose up against Russian occupation. Its people are struggling to develop their own form of democracy based in one of the largest parliament buildings in the world. Economic development has been slower than in other former Eastern Block nations, and Hungary remains one of Europe's poorer nations.

Hungary is worth a visit just for the general history and the arts, because this is a nation with deeply engrained passions for art, literature and opera. The capital city, Budapest, is really two cities joined by bridging the mighty Danube River. The "old city" is Buda, where most of the older historic buildings and monuments can be found. Pest was the industrial part that was founded to rebuild Buda (pest literally means oven, and there were plenty of these making bricks). The new, joined city is interesting in both of its halves, is easily accessible by air and rail, and has a very good public transport system that includes buses, trams and underground trains.

For those interested in medical education history, Budapest was the home of one of the profession's more recent iconic figures – Ignaz Semmelweis. A museum bearing his name is one of several sites of interest either near or within the Varhegy area (Area 1) of the city – surrounding Buda Palace (or castle) on the Burg (or hill).

12.1 Semmelweis Museum, Budapest

Ignaz Semmelweis was born in what is now the museum in 1818 into a large and wealthy Austrian family who were in Hungary during the Hapsburg Empire period. He initially studied law in Budapest, then later in Vienna, where he changed to medicine. This is also where he spent much of his early and middle career, specialising in obstetrics and surgery. He returned to Budapest as a professor at the Budapest Medical School in 1855.

CHAPTER 12

His great contribution to medical practice and education was his observation that women giving birth in a midwifery unit in Vienna had a much lower maternal death rate from puerperal fever than those in the medical unit. His theory was simple: doctors and medical students transmitted infections from outside the birthing suite. Unlike the midwives, who remained in the birthing suite, doctors and medical students moved all over the hospital, between inpatient wards, cadaver dissections, operating theatres and the birthing suites, but did not wash their hands thoroughly, thereby introducing infections to the almost sterile environment of the birthing suite. Similar discussions have resulted from the recent COVID-19 pandemic. This now obvious deduction was rejected by his medical colleagues as lunacy, and hand washing practices changed slowly, even though a trial of compulsory hand washing reduced maternal deaths by more than half. Semmelweis spent much of his life defending himself and promoting hand washing before contact with patients in the birthing suite and operating theatre and stopping patients with infections being nursed adjacent to women who had just had a normal birth.

This museum is almost the ideal regional medical history museum, because it has exhibitions of material summarising developments from ancient times through to the nineteenth century. There is coverage of ancient South American, Arab, Greek, Roman, medieval and Renaissance medicine, providing a brief but interesting summary of the major developments. Most of the collection is from the nineteenth century, reflecting developments in Hungary and, to a lesser extent, the Czech Republic, Slovakia and Austria, which were all part of the Hapsburg Empire.

Another pleasing feature of the museum is its juxtaposition of history, art and literature. There are some key manuscripts (Avicenna, Hippocrates, Galen and Maimonides) as well as a range of central European textbooks from the nineteenth century. The art collection is a combination of "mainstream" art by local doctors to medical topics such as consultations and clinical examinations.

For those interested in clinical skills development, there is a reasonable range of instruments used in clinical practice, including old weighing machines and sterilisers. A small range of Italian-made, full-scale wax models is also on display, and one room is a reconstruction of the original "Holy Ghost" apothecary, which dispensed medicines in the eighteenth and nineteenth centuries both directly to the public and on medical prescription.

Each display has descriptions in both English and Hungarian, so the material is accessible to English speakers. The museum staff were very helpful, although they speak much better German than English.

Further reading

Kapronczay, K. *Semmelweis*. Semmelweiss Museum, Budapest, 2004.

Location: Apród Utca 1-3, Budapest. This is at the southern base of the Burg.

Easiest access: The nearest tram lines are 19 and 61, but the walk from the commercial centre on the Pest side is just 15 minutes across the old suspension bridge (Erzsébet Híd).

Website: semmelweismuseum.hu/

General interest to medical history:		★★★★☆	
Relevance to medical education history:		★★★☆☆	
Ease of access:		★★★★☆	
Tourists	X	*Researchers*	

12.2. Golden Eagle Apothecary, Budapest

This small museum is managed by the Semmelweis Museum and is fifteen minutes' walk up the Castle Hill to the northern end, in the "civilian" area of the Burg. It was the original site of an herbal preparation laboratory in the fifteenth century and then later the Golden Eagle Apothecary. In Hungary, homeopathic medicine was popular with the people and apothecaries were a strong profession, although by the nineteenth century they were working more closely with doctors as community healers and the source of medicines.

There are displays of measuring, weighing, mixing and cooking apparatus, and a display of the wide range of plant and animal products that were included in medicines. There must have been some bizarre combinations, a bit like those spoken of in fairy tales! Unfortunately for foreigners, here all information is in Hungarian, so some of the information is not accessible to speakers of other languages.

Location: Tárnok Utca 18, Varhegy, Budapest.

Easiest access: At the northern end of the Burg, close to the Matyas church. The Number 22 bus goes up and down between the Burg and the Moskva tram and train station area.

Website: semmelweismuseum.hu/

General interest to medical history:		★★★☆☆	
Relevance to medical education history:		★★☆☆☆	
Ease of access:		★★★★☆	
Tourists	X	*Researchers*	X

12.3. Burg Labyrinth, Budapest

While in the Burg area it is also worth a brief look at the vast underground maze of corridors and chambers developed from the original limestone caves within the Burg. This has been used over several centuries as haven from battles. Of medical interest is an area used during the 1939–44 war as a "safe" hospital deep beneath a city that was almost destroyed (again!). There is not much to see, but enough to provoke the imagination of what it must have been like to work there.

Location: Úri Utca 9, Varhegy, Budapest. This is in the centre of the "civilian" Burg area on top of the hill. There is also an entrance/exit on the western side of the Burg, halfway up (or down) the zigzag access road.

Easiest access: Bus number 22 is a shuttle between the Burg and the Moskva Square tram and train station at the northern base of the Burg. If walking, try climbing the impressive stairway up from the riverbank, but only if you are very fit.

Website: budacastlebudapest.com/labyrinth-under-the-castle-hill/

General interest to medical history:		★★☆☆☆
Relevance to medical education history:		★☆☆☆☆
Ease of access:		★★★☆☆
Tourists	X	*Researchers*

CHAPTER 13:
THE NETHERLANDS

The Netherlands has in more recent times been one of the major international centres for research and development in medical education, with the relatively young University of Maastricht leading the way. However, the Netherlands can also claim a major role in the early development of medical education, because the University of Leiden pioneered the notion of clinical teaching much earlier than other European medical schools.

The origin of the university is a fascinating story. The port town was besieged by the Spanish in 1573 for a year and suffered terrible losses. Because the defence prevented the Spanish from taking over the whole region of the southern Netherlands, a grateful William of Orange offered the town the choice of either ten years of no taxes or a university; the town chose the latter. The university adopted the town's love of freedom from external control; it was not under religious authority and became famous for freedom of speech. Leiden University has developed as a strong research university, with a record of scholarship that matches many of the older, more traditional universities such as Cambridge, just across the water. Leiden itself is well worth a visit, as it is a compact university town with several museums, open air restaurants and interesting things to see. Tourism is big business, so everything is laid out in a well signposted and easily walkable route around and across the many canals. One museum celebrates the famous local artist, Rembrandt, but the main focus of this book is the Museum Boerhaave.

13.1. Museum Boerhaave, Leiden

The Museum Boerhaave pays homage to the developments in science and medicine in Leiden University. The medical school was planned soon after the university was established, and the early academic staff came from Padova. The museum is housed in the original medical school building, where a small clinical teaching unit was opened in 1636 in the St Cecilia Hospital. This was a revolutionary move within Europe, as medical education elsewhere remained largely theoretical, with no patient contact. Here students would learn medicine in a more integrated manner, with both theoretical instruction and bedside teaching from clinical professors and contact with patients. Interestingly, the current medical school at the University of Leiden is now one of the more conservative in the Netherlands, educationally speaking, as the local priority is biomedical scientific research. Perhaps because of this focus, the exhibition is much broader than medicine, and includes broader scientific and technical discoveries.

About half of the collection is directly relevant to medicine, and most of that has a focus on medical science and technology. While the entire exhibition is of course interesting, there are four sections that are particularly relevant to medical education. The first is a reconstruction of the original anatomy demonstration theatre, a small round theatre, where learners could observe human dissection. The structure is in concept similar to the Padova theatre but is much smaller. A visitor can walk around the outside and see clearly how it functioned. The second is a limited collection of full-colour wax anatomical models that were made locally. These differ from the Italian models seen elsewhere, in that not all are life size. However, some are in large scale to demonstrate to learners the details of smaller parts of the human body.

The third part relevant to medical education is a room that focuses on the Dutch development of medical specialties during the nineteenth century. Much of this appears to be related to the ability of Leiden academics to produce new machinery to assist with eye and ear surgery. There is also a large display of a wide range of locally developed surgical and obstetric instruments. The final part is an unusual collection of Zander machines, named after their inventor. These are large machines in which humans could sit or stand, while single muscle groups could be exercised repetitively, such as in stroke recovery. For a while they were a very popular form of physiotherapy in the Netherlands.

Location: Lange Sint Agnietenstraat 10, Leiden.

Easiest access: A 10-minute walk through the old city centre from Leiden Central Station (30 mins from Amsterdam).

Website: www.museumboerhaave.nl

General interest to medical history:		★★★☆☆	
Relevance to medical education history:		★★☆☆☆	
Ease of access:		★★★☆☆	
Tourists	X	Researchers	

CHAPTER 14:
DENMARK

The Scandinavian countries are not often thought of in the history of medical education, but they played their part. There were strong links and parallels with the German system of medical education, although academic development followed a unique path that combined elements of Italian, French, Dutch and English experiences. As formal medical education expanded across Europe, and the battles between factions within the Church split Christianity into Catholic and Protestant groups, so too did Denmark have to establish its own university system, rather than rely on sending its young scholars a substantial distance to attend other universities. In Denmark, the development of a university followed quite soon after early developments in Germany and the Netherlands.

14.1. Medical Museum, Copenhagen

This museum contains a rather eclectic collection of equipment, photographs and other memorabilia relevant to the development of medical practice over three centuries in Denmark. As elsewhere in Europe, apothecaries, surgeons and physicians had separate origins and histories, although this museum includes material relevant to all three. The University of Copenhagen was established

CHAPTER 14

in 1479 – the second oldest in northern Europe – with faculties of law, philosophy and medicine. Until then Copenhagen's doctors were trained elsewhere, usually in Italy. One such medical practitioner, Jesper Henriksen, was the first university Rector. Meanwhile, the local Company of Barber Surgeons was formed in 1505 and they grew in strength. In 1787 they formed the Academy of Surgeons and introduced more formal training for members, achieving equivalent status to physicians.

In 1842 the Academy of Surgeons merged with the Faculty of Medicine to offer a combined training program and the Academy Hall became the main site of medical education for the University. The teaching complex included a demonstration lecture theatre, as well as clinical services such as an apothecary and operating theatres. It was next door to the main women's hospital – the Royal Frederik Maternity Hospital – regarded as one of the best women's teaching hospitals in northern Europe.

The museum is within the original Academy of Surgery Hall and holds interesting displays relevant to public health, surgery and psychiatry. The public health display includes graphs plotting the local outbreaks of the Spanish Flu (1918–21) and polio (1951–3), and information about earlier outbreaks of leprosy, syphilis, smallpox, tuberculosis and the plague. The psychiatry section includes some amazing restraining devices that provide insight to psychiatric practice of the era. Along with straitjackets and models of solitary confinement cells, there is a commode chair in which a deranged person could be locked. In keeping with the origins of the building, the strength of the museum is the surgical displays that reflect the emergence of new surgical specialties during the last 150 years – orthopaedic, ophthalmological, ear, nose and throat, dental and gynaecological. There are old anaesthetic machines and surgical equipment, and of course the demonstration lecture theatre that is still used for research dissertation presentations. Some gems include an early ophthalmoscope from about 1850, clear instructions, with models, on how to amputate limbs, and early models of the inner ear used to instruct surgeons.

Choose visiting times carefully. English language tours can be booked, and an English language guidebook is available. Displays have dual Danish/English labels and I had little difficulty working things out. While in Copenhagen also visit the original university building near the Town Hall Square – a magnificent medieval Baronial Hall.

Location: Bredogade 62, Copenhagen.

Easiest access: Bus number 6 or 29 from city centre.

Website: www.museion.ku.dk/en/

General interest to medical history:		★★★☆☆	
Relevance to medical education history:		★★★☆☆	
Ease of access:		★★★☆☆	
Tourists	X	Researchers	

BIBLIOGRAPHY

2001 Summer Dream Editions. *Kos.* Stelios Kontaratos, Athens, 2001.

Encyclopaedia Judaica. Encyclopaedia Judaica; Macmillan Jerusalem, 1971.

Arnold, C. *Bedlam: London and its Mad.* Simon and Schuster, London, 2008.

Bell, E. Moberly. *Storming the Citadel: the Rise of the Woman Doctor.* Constable, London, 1953.

Blandy, J.P. and Lumley, J.S.P. *The Royal College of Surgeons of England: 200 Years of History at the Millennium.* Royal College of Surgeons of England, London, 2000.

Boulton, T. *The Association of Anaesthetists of Great Britain and Ireland 1932-1992 and the Development of the Specialty of Anaesthesia: Sixty Years of Progress and Achievement in the Context of Scientific, Political and Social Change.* Association of Anaesthetists of Great Britain and Ireland, London, 1999.

Chadwick, J. and Mann, W.N. *The Medical Works of Hippocrates.* Blackwell Scientific Publications, Oxford, 1950.

Clark, G. *A History of the Royal College of Physicians of London.* Clarendon Press, Oxford, 1964.

Coar, Thomas, translator. *The Aphorisms of Hippocrates.* 1822. Reprint Classics of Medicine Library, Gryphon Editions, Birmingham, Alabama, 1995.

Cohn, S. K. *The Black Death Transformed: Disease and Culture in early Renaissance Europe*. Hodder Education, London, 2003.

Cuenant, E. Bonnel, F., Bonnet, H., Charlot, C., Lorblanchet, H. and Vial, M. *Médecine, Art et Histoire à Montpellier*. Sauramps Editions, Montpellier, 2002.

Davidson, H.E. *Moses Maimonides. The Man and His Works*. Oxford University Press, New York, 2004.

Duncum, B. *The Development of Inhalation Anaesthesia*. Oxford University Press, 1947. Reprinted Royal Society of Medicine Press, London, 1994.

Ead, Hamed A. Averroes as a Physician. www.levity.com/alchemy/islam21.html

Filer, J. *Egyptian Bookshelf: Disease*. British Museum Press, London, 1995.

Gerber, Jane S. T*he Jews of Spain. A History of the Sephardic Experience*. Free Press, New York, 1992.

Goldsworthy, P.D. and McFarlane A.C. "Howard Florey, Alexander Fleming and the fairy tale of penicillin." *Medical Journal of Australia*, vol 176, no. 4, 2002. eMJA. www.mja.com.au/public/issues/176_04180202/gol10735.html. Accessed March 2004.

Guthrie, D. *A History of Medicine*. Thomas Nelson and Sons, London, 1945. Reprinted 1960.

Haeger, K. *An Illustrated History of Surgery*. Harold Stark Medical, London, 1989.

Hameed, H.A and Avicenna. *Avicenna's Tract on Cardiac Drugs and Essays on Arab Cardiotherapy*. Hamdard Foundation Press, Karachi, 1983.

Hunting, P. *A History of the Society of Apothecaries*. The Society of Apothecaries, London, 1998.

Kapronczay, K. *Semmelweis*. Semmelweiss Museum, Budapest, 2004.

Lock, S, Last, J.M. and Dunea, G. (Eds). *The Oxford Illustrated Companion to Medicine*. Oxford University Press, 2001.

McManus, I.C. *Right Hand, Left Hand*. Weidenfeld and Nicolson, London, 2002.

Ozaydin, Zuhal. "Some landmarks in the history of medicine in Istanbul (Materials, Books, Documents, Periodicals and Buildings)." *Journal of the International Society for the History of Islamic Medicine*, vol. 3. 2004, pp. 26–29.

Parente, P.P. *The Regimen of Health of The Medical School of Salerno*. Vantage Press, New York, 1967.

Puschmann, T. and Hare, E.H. *A History of Medical Education*. [Translated and edited by E.H. Hare] Facsimile of 1891 ed. Hafner, New York 1966.

Rawcliffe, Carole. *Medicine and Society in Later Medieval England*. Sutton Publishing Ltd, London, 1995.

Robinson, V. *Pathfinders in Medicine*. Medical Life Press, New York, 1929.

Sari N. "Educating the Ottoman physician." *History of Medicine Studies*, 1988; pp. 40–64. www.muslimheritage.com/topics/default.cfm?Article ID=632.

Sarton, George. *Galen of Pergamon*. University of Kansas Press, Lawrence, Kansas, 1954.

Shapiro, John. *The Jewish 100. A Ranking of the Most Influential Jews of All Time*. Citadel Press, New York, 1994.

Sigerist, H.E. *A History of Medicine*. Oxford University Press, New York, 1961.

Singer, C. and Underwood, E.A. *A Short History of Medicine*. 2nd ed., Oxford University Press, London, 1962.

Springer, C. "Cos and Hippocrates. A Historical Revision." *British Medical Journal*, 16 October, 1943, vol. 2, p. 492.

Walsh, Mary Roth. *"Doctors Wanted: No Women Need Apply". Sexual Barriers in the Medical Profession, 1835–1975*. Yale University Press, New Haven, 1977.

www.ingramcontent.com/pod-product-compliance
Lightning Source LLC
Chambersburg PA
CBHW070306010526
44107CB00056B/2503